Radia Benyahia

Breast imaging of benign lesions in general practice

Radia Benyahia

Breast imaging of benign lesions in general practice

Essential guide to the diagnosis of benign breast lesions

ScienciaScripts

Imprint

Cover image: www.ingimage.com

This book is a translation from the original published under ISBN 978-620-6-71082-0.

Publisher:
Sciencia Scripts
is a trademark of
Dodo Books Indian Ocean Ltd. and OmniScriptum S.R.L publishing group

120 High Road, East Finchley, London, N2 9ED, United Kingdom
Str. Armeneasca 28/1, office 1, Chisinau MD-2012, Republic of Moldova, Europe
Managing Directors: Ieva Konstantinova, Victoria Ursu
info@omniscriptum.com

Printed at: see last page
ISBN: 978-620-8-53102-7

Contents

PREFACE

Breast Imaging of Negligible Lesions in General Practice is designed specifically for general practitioners to introduce them to the fundamental principles and practical applications of breast imaging in the diagnosis and follow-up of breast lesions.

Through this guide, we will explore the various imaging modalities such as mammography, breast ultrasound and MRI. They will learn not only how these techniques are used in clinical settings to assess and manage breast pathology, but also how they fit into an overall treatment plan for patients. This textbook aims to enrich their academic learning with practical knowledge that will prepare you for thoughtful and informed clinical interventions. The aim is to equip them with the tools they need to interpret imaging results competently and to collaborate effectively with radiologists and other specialists in patient care. We hope that this guide will serve as a cornerstone of their medical training and also stimulate their interest in radiology, a specialty which, although often operating behind the scenes, is indispensable to the accurate diagnosis and effective treatment of many medical conditions.

List of employees

Chahira Mazouzi, Senior Lecturer in Medical Oncology, CHU Bejaia.

Kamel Hail, senior lecturer in general surgery, Hôpital Mustapha, Algiers.

General

1. Introduction

Imaging exploration of benign breast lesions is the mainstay of the diagnostic process, complementing the clinical examination and in-depth questioning. It is used both for the initial identification of lesions and to determine their extent, and for monitoring patients after treatment.

2. Diagnosis

The diagnostic process always begins with a detailed clinical assessment, which may be followed imaging investigations. The latter may be initiated following the discovery of abnormalities during the clinical examination or as part of screening programmes, which target women between the ages of 40 and 70 for organised screening, or at any age for individual screening.

3. Medical imaging in the evaluation of breast tumours

The imaging procedure generally includes mammography, supplemented by ultrasound in cases of high breast density or in younger women. The formal diagnosis is made on the basis of histological analysis of biopsy samples, guided by the imaging results.

3.1. Mammography

Offered every two years to women aged between 50 and 74, mammography must cover both breasts and be based on bilateral comparisons and comparisons with previous images. It includes two views of each breast.

Mammograms are interpreted using the American College of Radiology's BI-RADS system, which classifies the results into seven categories to guide management:

1) Category 0: more information ;
2) Category 1: Mammography with no abnormalities ;
3) Category 2: Clearly benign abnormality ;
4) Category 3: Anomaly probably benign, requiring short-term follow-up;
5) Category 4: Suspicious lesion, histological verification recommended ;
6) Category 5: Lesion strongly suggestive of malignancy ;
7) Category 6: Malignancy confirmed by biopsy.

Cases classified in categories 1 and 2 may be re-read by a second radiologist for organised screening.

3.2. Mammary ultrasound

Used as a complementary examination, ultrasound enables lesions detected on mammography to be better characterised, particularly in women over 40, in the presence of dense breasts or when clinical abnormalities are not visible on mammography. It also plays a key role in guiding biopsies.

3.3. Mammary MRI

MRI is reserved for specific situations, such as screening patients at high genetic risk due to BRCA1 or BRCA2 mutations.

This multidimensional approach, combining clinical examination and imaging techniques, optimises the diagnosis and therapeutic strategy for breast tumours, while tailoring post-treatment follow-up to each patient.

CHAPTER 1

Imaging simple mammary cysts

1. Introduction

The mammary cyst is a frequent benign lesion, characterised by pockets or cavities filled with fluid, surrounded by a wall encapsulated within the breast tissue. They can occur at any age, but are more common in women aged between 30 and 50. Imaging plays an essential role in the assessment of breast cysts, an accurate diagnosis to be made and differentiating cysts from other breast lesions. This fact sheet focuses on the imaging features of simple cysts, helping to identify and manage them.

2. Epidemiology

High prevalence in women of childbearing age, decreasing after the menopause except in women on HRT (hormone replacement therapy). Can occur under hormonal influence.

3. Pathophysiology

Result of obstruction of the milk ducts, leading to accumulation of fluid. Not linked to an increased risk of breast cancer.

4. Clinical presentation

Often asymptomatic. May appear as a palpable, round or oval mass that is mobile and flexible. May cause mild discomfort or pain, particularly before menstruation.

1.1. Mammography

Mammography is one of the methods used to investigate cysts in women over the age of 40. The typical characteristics of a mammary cyst on mammography include :

1) A round or oval mass, well circumscribed with regular contours if the weft is fatty, masked if the weft is dense;
2) Low density or isodense in relation to surrounding breast tissue.

1.2. Ultrasound

Ultrasound is an imaging modality par excellence, and is used as the first line of defence in characterising breast cysts. The ultrasound characteristics of cysts include :

1) A well-defined anechogenic mass with a thin, regular wall;
2) Oval or rounded shape;
3) Reinforced post-acoustics (posterior reinforcement) due to the transmission of sound through the cyst fluid;

4) Anechoic, homogeneous with posterior reinforcement ... .

1.3. MRI (Magnetic Resonance Imaging)

MRI features of cysts include:

1) A well-defined mass with regular, circumscribed margins;
2) A high-intensity signal in the T2 sequence, indicating the presence of liquid;
3) A low-intensity signal in sequence T1 ;
4) No enhancement after injection of contrast medium.

6. Conclusion

Imaging plays an important role in the diagnosis of breast cysts. The combination of these imaging modalities makes it possible to establish a precise diagnosis and to differentiate cysts from other breast lesions, classifying them as ACR BI-RADS 2. The course of action is no surveillance and no further surveillance examinations.

7. References

1) Berg WA, Mendelson EB, et al. ACR BI-RADS® Ultrasound. In: ACR BI-RADS® Atlas, Breast Imaging Reporting and Data System. Reston, VA: American College of Radiology; 2013.

2) 2. American College of Radiology. Breast Imaging Reporting and Data System (BIRADS®). 5th ed. Reston, VA: American College of Radiology; 2013.

3) 3. Morris EA, Comstock CE, et al. ACR BI-RADS® Magnetic Resonance Imaging. In: ACR BI-RADS® Atlas, Breast Imaging Reporting and Data system.

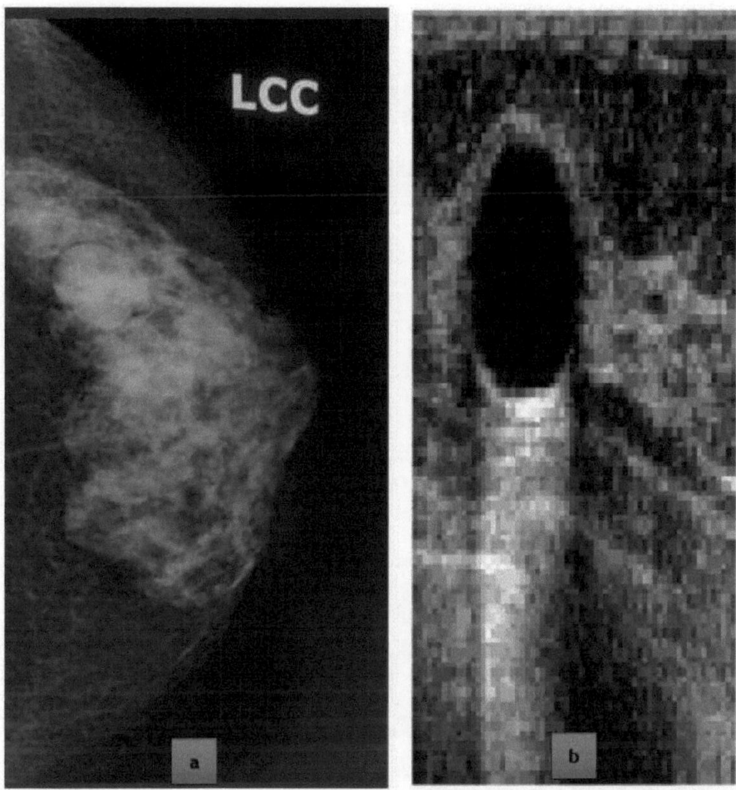

Figure 1. a. Circumscribed, rounded mass, isodence, homogeneous, possibly related to a simple cyst on mammography.

b. Circumscribed mass with anechogenic content and posterior enhancement suggestive of a Simple cyst on ultrasound

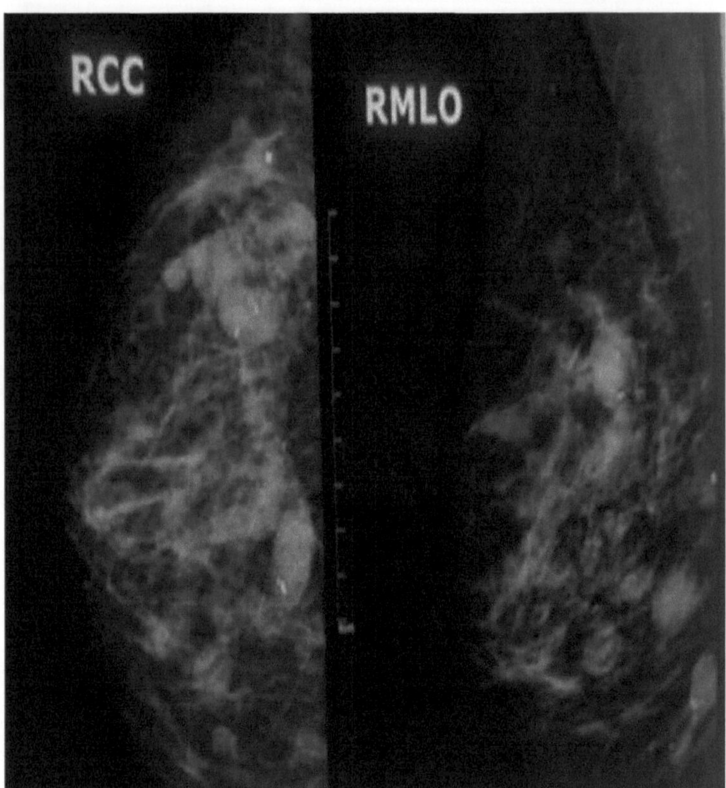

Figure 2. right mammogram, frontal and external oblique views: circumscribed, scattered iso-dense masses, some of which have peripheral popcorn calcifications in association with cystic dystrophy.

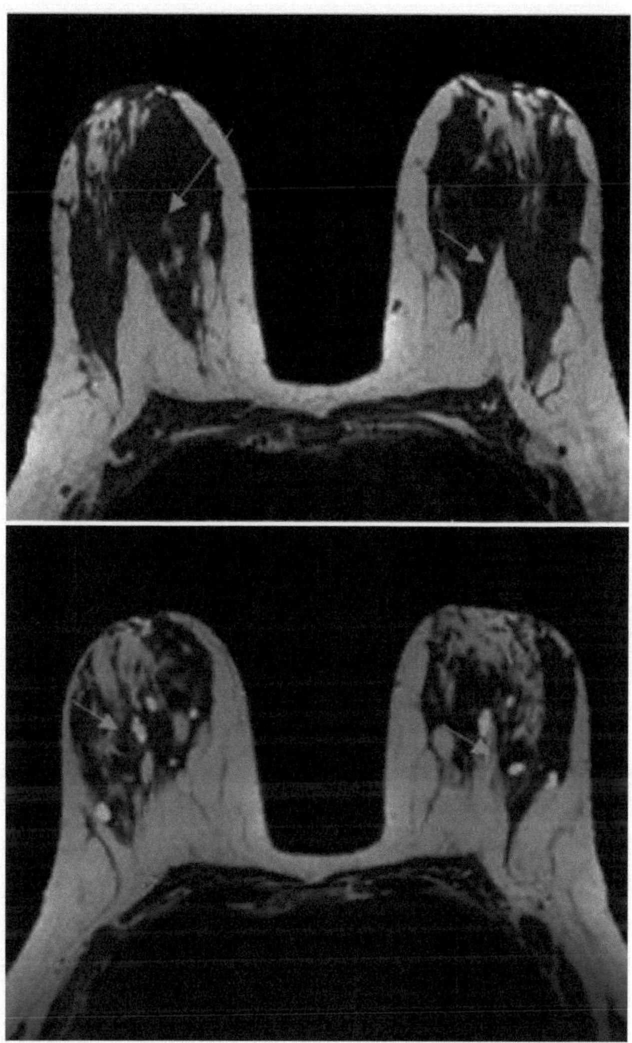

Figure 3. Simple and bilateral cyst dystrophies on MRI, in T1 hyposignal(a), T2 hyper signal(b)

III. Imaging of complicated breast cysts

1. Introduction

Complicated mammary cysts represent an evolution of simple cysts, characterised by internal changes that may raise diagnostic doubts. Complicated breast cysts are cystic lesions with atypical features or significant changes in their contents. Although they remain mostly benign, their appearance on imaging can sometimes mimic that of malignant lesions, necessitating a different course of action to that for simple cysts.

2. Epidemiology

Less common than simple cysts. Can occur at any age, but more common in women of childbearing age and in the peri-menopause.

3. Pathophysiology

Often result from haemorrhage or infection of a simple cyst, or the presence of cellular debris, leading to complex ultrasound features.

Not associated with a risk of cancer, but require in-depth caracterisation to exclude malignant pathology.

4. Clinical presentation

May be asymptomatic but more often present as a palpable mass. May cause a sensation of heaviness or mild pain, particularly if the cyst is inflamed or infected.

These cysts may be associated with clinical symptoms such as pain, inflammation or worrying radiological features.

Imaging plays an essential role in the assessment of complicated breast cysts, enabling these lesions to be differentiated from other breast pathologies. This fact sheet provides an in-depth understanding of the imaging techniques used to assess complicated breast cysts.

1.1. Mammography

Radiological features of complicated breast cysts on mammography include:

1) An increase in the density of the cyst in relation to the surrounding breast tissue;

2) The presence of calcifications, particularly coarse or pleomorphic calcifications;

3) A cyst that changes significantly in size, shape or density during radiological follow-up.

1.2. Ultrasound

Ultrasound is an essential imaging modality for characterising complicated breast cysts. Sonographic features of complicated cysts include:

1) A mass with circumscribed contours, sometimes blurred;
2) A combination of solid and cystic components;
3) A thickened wall due to inflammation;
4) Mixed echogenicity with internal echoes, fine echoes representing debris particles or solid echoes;
5) The presence of complex internal structures, such as septa or solid echoes;
6) No posterior reinforcement.

1.3. MRI (Magnetic Resonance Imaging) :

MRI features of complicated cysts include:

1) Defined contours ;
2) Heterogeneous signals on T1- and T2-weighted sequences, indicating a solid component or haemorrhage;
3) Contrast after injection of contrast medium ;
4) The presence of raised septa.

6. Conclusion

Imaging plays an important role in the evaluation of complicated breast cysts, enabling these lesions to be differentiated from other breast pathologies with similar characteristics. Mammography, ultrasound and MRI are complementary modalities that provide detailed information on the nature, composition and vascularisation of cysts. Complicated cysts are classified as ACR BI-RADS 3. Monitoring in 4 months is recommended.

Follow-up

Complicated breast cysts that are asymptomatic, stable over time and have benign radiological features can be monitored regularly with follow-up imaging examinations.

Cysts that are symptomatic, increasing in size or have worrying radiological features may require puncture or aspiration of the cyst contents to relieve symptoms and confirm the diagnosis.

7. References

1) Gallego, G. (2005). "Nódulo Palpable de Mama. " *Revista Colombiana de Obstetricia y Ginecología*.

2) Heath, C. B. (2010). "Breast cyst aspiration. "In Primary Care Procedures in Women's Health. https: //doi. org/10. 1007/978-0-387-76604-1_19

3) Jackson, V. P., & Bassett, L. W. (1998). "Breast sonography. "Breast Disease. https: //doi. org/10. 3233/BD-1998-103-408

4) Early Breast Cancer Trialists' Collaborative Group (EBCTCG). (2005). "Effects

of chemotherapy and hormonal therapy for early breast cancer on recurrence and 15-year survival: an overview of the randomised trials. "The Lancet. https: //doi. org/10. 1016/S0140-6736(05)66544-0
5) American Cancer Society (2016). "Breast Cancer; What is breast cancer?" https: //doi. org/10. 1002/9780470041000. cedt005

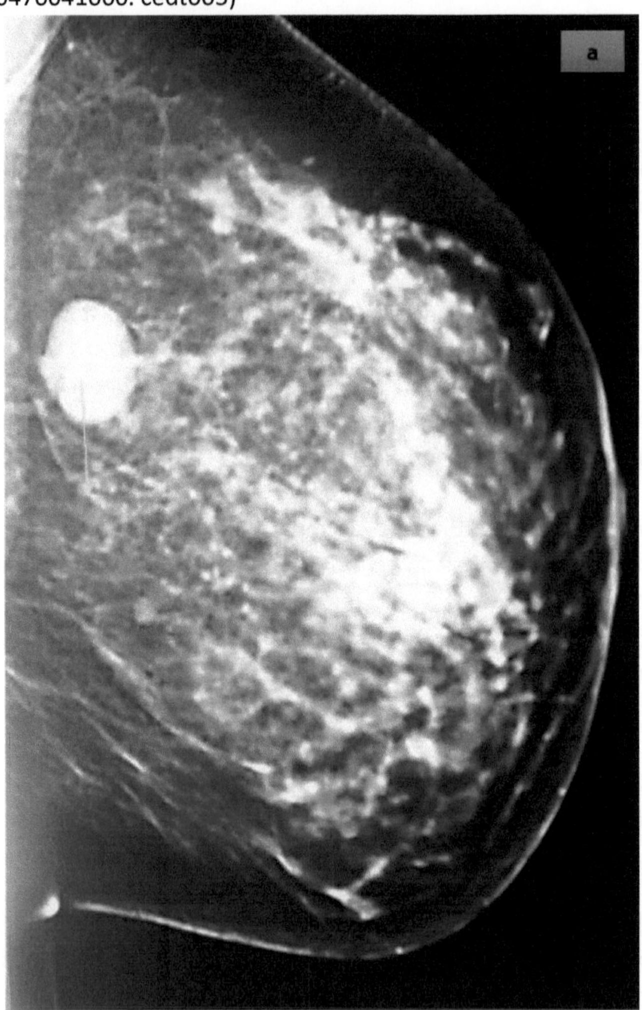

Figure 1. a. Mammogram, left oblique view: circumscribed, rounded mass of homogeneous high density in the upper quadrant.

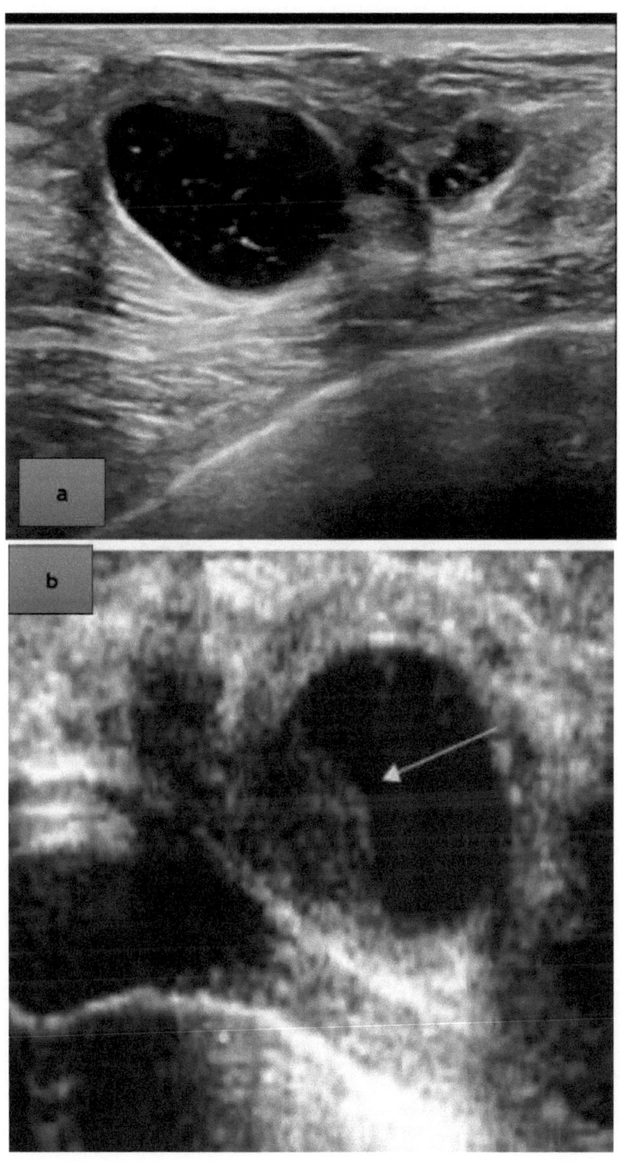
a
b

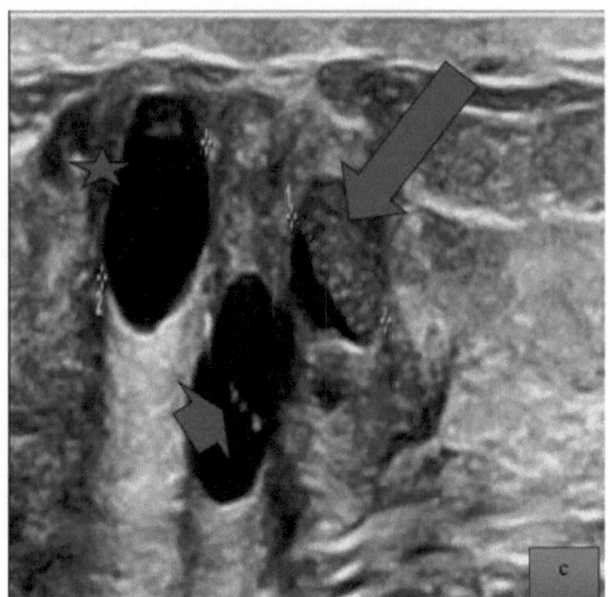

Figure 2. breast ultrasound a. Complicated cyst, with anechogenic content, finely echogenic. b. Complicated cyst, with anechogenic content, finely echogenic downstage. c. Complicated cyst, with anechogenic content (star), finely echogenic throughout (arrow), septated (arrowhead).

IV. Imaging a cluster of cysts embedded in the breast tissue

1. Introduction

Clusters of cysts embedded in the breast tissue represent a particular type of cystic lesion, characterised by the presence of multiple cysts grouped together within the breast tissue. Also known as juvenile papillomatosis, it occurs in women under the age of 30. It is a localised fibrocystic dystrophy. This entity can pose a diagnostic challenge, particularly in distinguishing benign cystic clusters from solid lesions or cystic formations with malignant potential. Accurate imaging assessment is therefore essential for appropriate management.

2. Etiology

Mammary cysts are benign lesions, often resulting from fibrocystic changes in the breast. Clusters of cysts may be associated with hormonal changes, trauma or inflammatory processes. Clinical expression may be either :

- A palpable mass;
- An irregular, sensitive cupboard.

3. Imaging methods

3.1. Mammography

Clusters of cysts may appear as areas of increased density with or without well-defined contours, making them difficult to identify in some cases, especially in women with dense breast tissue. Cysts may not be clearly differentiated from solid masses. Mammography may reveal microcalcifications (in three out of four cases), within an overdensity that is poorly defined or poly-lobed.

3.2. Mammary ultrasound

Best modality for visualising cyst clusters, showing well circumscribed anechogenic formations with posterior sound enhancement, within focal glandular tissue. Cysts can vary in size and shape.

3.3. Magnetic Resonance Imaging (MRI) of the breast

Cysts show a hyperintense signal in T2 and are generally hypointense in T1, with no enhancement after injection of gadolinium, except for the walls or septa which are thickened. Used for further evaluation, particularly when the results of ultrasound and mammography are ambiguous or when the presence of solid components is suspected.

4. Care and Support

Ultrasound monitoring is often sufficient for typically benign cyst clusters, with periodic follow-up to monitor any changes.

> **Biopsy:** Indicated if atypical features are present or if a clear distinction with malignant lesions cannot be made;

> **Surgery:** Rarely necessary, except in the case of significant symptoms or aesthetic concerns on the part of the patient.

5. Conclusion

Clusters of cysts embedded in the breast tissue are generally benign, classified as BI- RADS 3 by the ACR, but accurate characterisation by imaging is important to exclude malignancy. Breast ultrasound plays a central role in the initial assessment, supplemented by mammography and, if necessary, MRI for further analysis. The management of these lesions depends on their imaging characteristics, the presence of symptoms, and the patient's preferences, favouring a personalised approach to the management of cystic breast masses.

6. References

1) Gallego, G. (2005). "Nódulo Palpable de Mama. "Revista Colombiana de Obstetricia y Ginecología*.

2) Heath, C. B. (2010). "Breast cyst aspiration. "In Primary Care Procedures in Women's Health. [DOI: 10. 1007/978-0-387-76604 1_19](https: //doi. org/10. 1007/978-0-387-76604-1_19)

3) Jackson, V. P., & Bassett, L. W. (1998). "Breast sonography. "Breast Disease. [DOI: 10. 3233/BD-1998-103-408](https: //doi. org/10. 3233/BD-1998-103-408)

4) Early Breast Cancer Trialists' Collaborative Group (EBCTCG). (2005). "Effects of chemotherapy and hormonal therapy for early breast cancer on recurrence and 15-year survival: an overview of the randomised trials. "The Lancet. [DOI: 10. 1016/S0140-6736(05)66544-0](https: //doi. org/10. 1016/S0140-6736(05)66544- 0)

5) American Cancer Society (2016). "Breast Cancer; What is breast cancer?" [DOI: 10. 1002/9780470041000. cedt005](https://doi . org/10. 1002/9780470041000. cedt005)

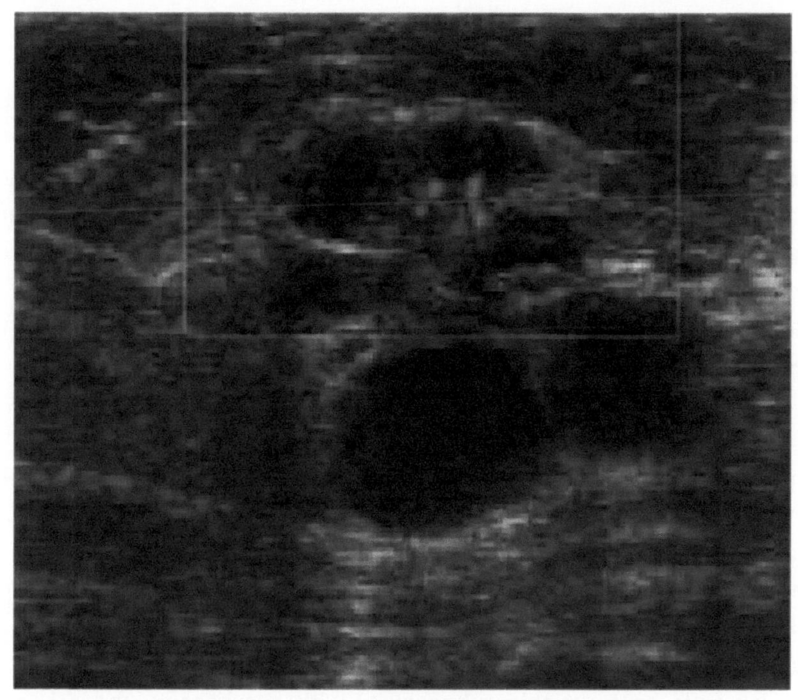

Fig 1. Breast ultrasound: cluster of microcysts in a focal hyperechoic area (juvenile papillomatosis).

V. Imaging complex mammary cysts

1. Introduction

Complex breast cysts are lesions with blurred contours and heterogeneous internal features on imaging. They are distinguished from simple cysts by the presence of thick septae or intracystic nodules, and can sometimes pose a diagnostic challenge by mimicking malignant lesions, requiring an ultrasound-guided microbiopsy directed at the suspected area including the cyst wall. Placement of an intra-lesional clip is essential because of the risk of disappearance of the lesion, particularly small lesions *(*< 7mm), and in the event of planned neoadjuvant chemotherapy.

2. Imaging methods

2.1. Mammography

Complex cysts may appear as dense masses with or without calcifications. The septa or wall thickenings are not visible.

2.2. Mammary ultrasound

The method of choice for evaluating breast cysts, distinguishing between solid and fluid lesions and guiding biopsy procedures. Allows visualization of the liquid nature of the lesion, septations, wall thickening, and intracystic nodules. Complex cysts have variable echogenicity with anechogenic and echogenic areas.

2.3. Magnetic Resonance Imaging (MRI) of the breast

Offers superior contrast resolution, allowing detailed assessment of the internal features of complex cysts, including the presence of solid components. It is used for cases that are indeterminate on ultrasound or to assess the extent of disease in patients with suspicious or malignant lesions.

3. Diagnostic criteria

➢ In favour of benignity: cysts with fine septae, without solid nodules or significant wall thickening ;

➢ Suspicion of malignancy: Presence of solid nodules, irregular thickening of the wall, or signs of abnormal vascularisation on Doppler ultrasound.

4. Care and Support

➢ **Monitoring:** Benign complex cysts can be monitored by ultrasound at regular intervals;

➢ **Biopsy:** Lesions with suspicious or undetermined features require biopsy under ultrasound guidance to rule out malignancy.

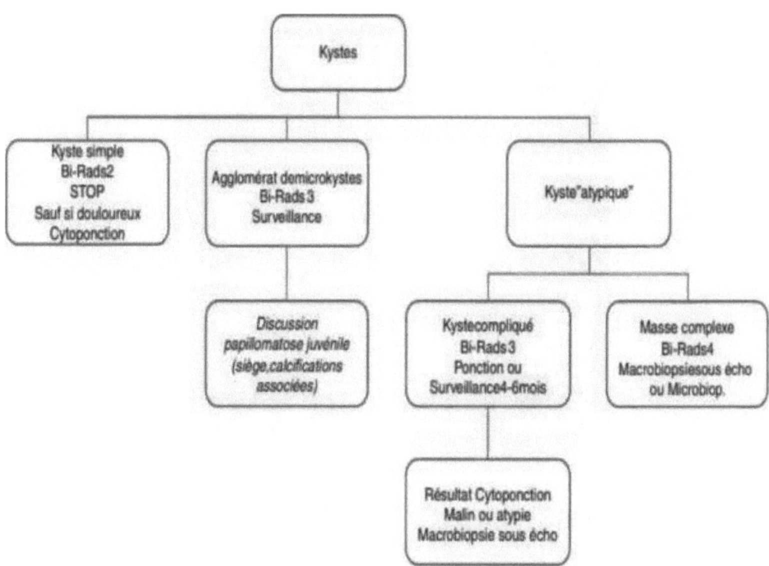

5. References

1) Candelaria RP, Hwang L, Bouchard RR, Whitman GJ. Breast ultrasound: current concepts. Semin Ultrasound CT MR 2013;34(3): 213-25.

2) Youk JH, Gweon HM, Son EJ, Han KH, Kim JA. Diagnostic value of commercially available shear-wave elastography for breast cancers: integration into BI-RADS classification with subcategories of category 4. Eur Radiol 2013;23(10): 2695- 704.

3) Berg WA, Campassi CI, Ioffe OB. Cystic lesions of the breast: sonographic-pathologic correlation. Radiology 2003;227(1): 183-91. Cystic masses complexities in breast ultrasound 185

4) Trop I, Dugas A, David J, El Khoury M, Boileau JF, Larouche N, et al. Breast abscesses: evidence-based algorithms for diagnosis, management, and follow-up. Radiographics 2011;31(6): 1683-99

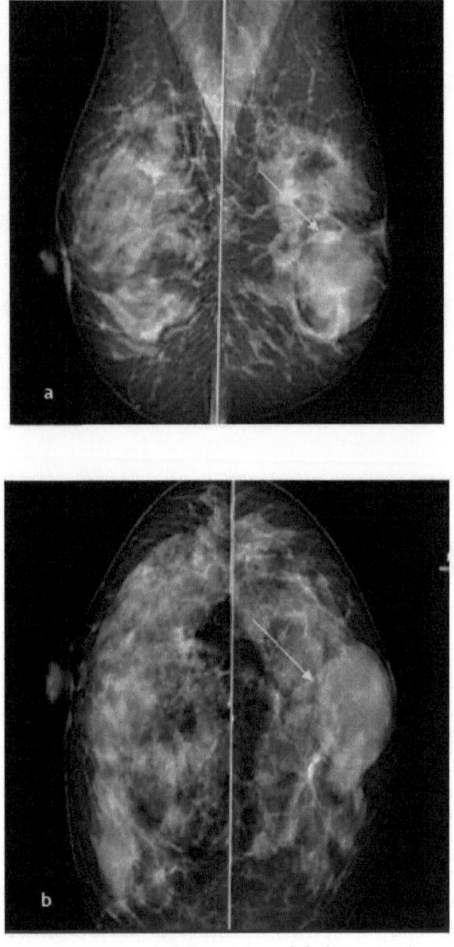

Figure 1: Bilateral mammogram: external oblique views (a), faces. Isodense mass of the left IMQ, roughly rounded, circumscribed, homogeneous (b).

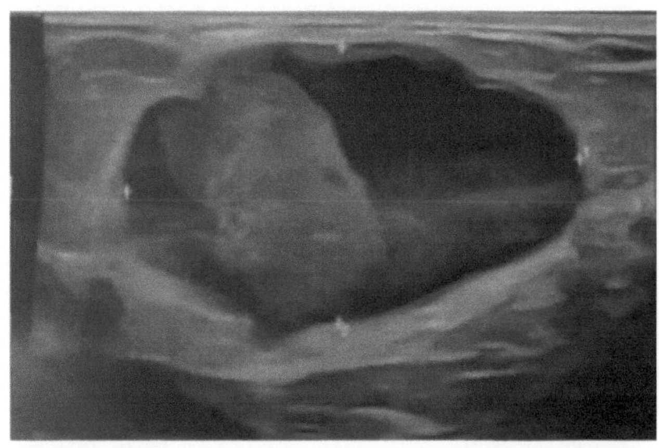

Figure 2. breast ultrasound scan. Complex lobulated mass with circumscribed solid-cystic contours with cystic predominance

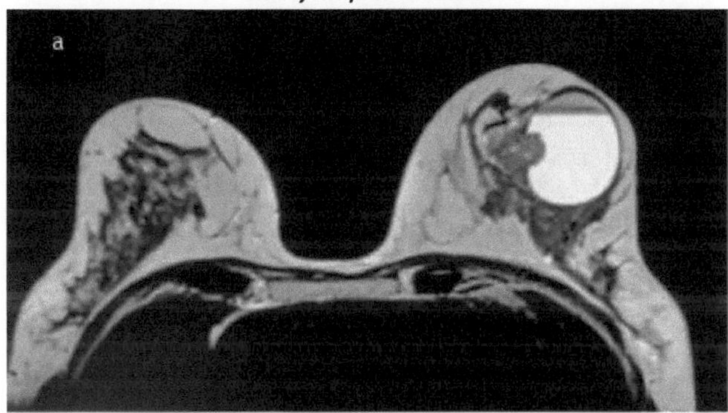

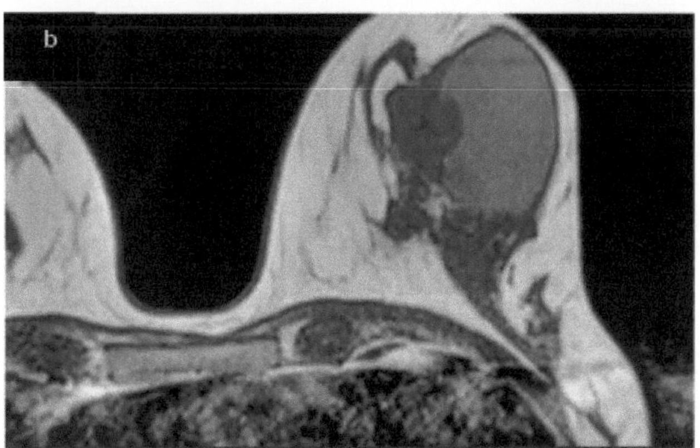

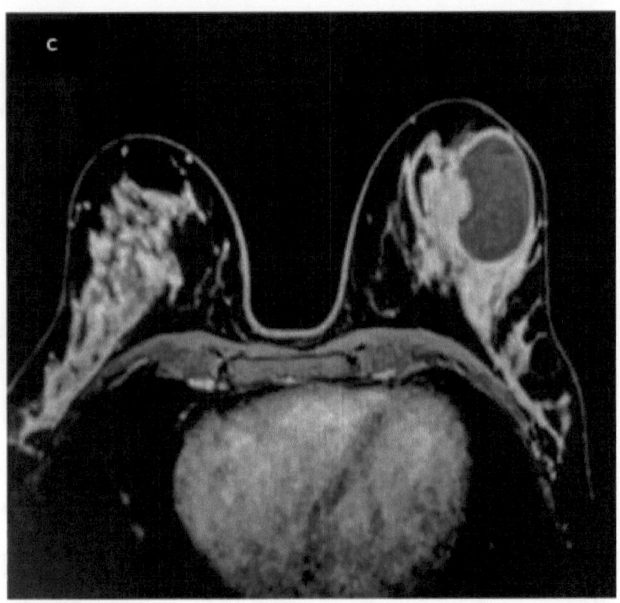

Figure 3. MRI of the breast, axial sections. a. T2-weighted sequential: left breast soli do cystic masses in heterogeneous T2 hypersignal; b. Sequenced T1-weighted T1 hyposignal; c. Heterogeneous enhancement of the fleshy component and thickening of the peripheral wall

VI. Imaging mammary galactoceles

1. Introduction

Mammary galactoceles are benign lesions of the breast that form as a result of the accumulation of milk in the milk ducts, generally due to the obstruction of a galactophore duct. They occur most often in women who are breastfeeding or after weaning. This fact sheet covers the essential imaging features of galactoceles to help identify and manage them.

2. Epidemiology

Predominantly in post-partum women, those who are breastfeeding or after weaning. Can occur at any age during the reproductive period, but is more common in young mothers.

3. Pathophysiology

A galactocele forms as a result of obstruction of a milk duct, leading to an accumulation of milk. The composition of the fluid may change over time, becoming more oily or thicker, which affects its appearance on imaging.

4. Clinical presentation

Often discovered incidentally or when palpating a soft, mobile, painless mass. May cause slight discomfort, but generally asymptomatic.

5. Imaging

Imaging plays an essential role in the evaluation of breast galactoceles, particularly when there is clinical suspicion.

5.1. Mammography

Mammography is often used as the primary imaging modality to assess breast galactoceles. Radiological features of mammographic galactoceles include:

1) A well-circumscribed mass, often round or oval, with circumscribed contours;

2) Variable radiological density, depending on the concentration of milky fluid inside the galactocele;

3) They may appear as well-defined lesions, but the density may vary according to the composition of the contents;

4) Fat-rich galactoceles may appear radiolucent, while those with a denser content will be radiopaque;

5) Absence of significant calcifications;

Mammary galactoceles can be located in any part of the breast, but they are often observed in the superior-external quadrants and in the retroarolar region.

5.2. Ultrasound

Breast ultrasound is an essential imaging modality for characterising breast galactoceles. Sonographic features of galactoceles include:

1) A well-circumscribed mass, often anechoic, with circumscribed contours;

2) Thick, hyperechoic walls in the periphery, corresponding to the fibrous capsule of the galactocele;

3) May have internal liquid-liquid levels or floating internal echoes depending on content separation.

5.3. MRI (Magnetic Resonance Imaging)

Breast MRI is a sensitive imaging modality for detecting and characterising breast galactoceles, but its use is less common than mammography and ultrasound. MRI features include:

1) A well-circumscribed mass with smooth contours. Continuous tubular structures with a nipple orientation and water or fat content can be seen;

2) A signal that varies according to the concentration of milky fluid inside the galactocele;

3) No significant enhancement after injection of contrast medium in the absence of clinical signs of inflammation.

6. Conclusion

Galactoceles are benign lesions associated with breastfeeding, characterised by distinct imaging presentations that reflect their content. An informed diagnostic approach and conservative management are often sufficient, minimising discomfort for the patient while avoiding unnecessary interventions.

7. References

1) Park YH, Lee YH, Kwon TH. Ultrasonographic findings of breast diseases during pregnancy and lactating period. J Korean Radiol Soc. 1995;33(3): 443-7. [Google Scholar]

2) Amr SS, Sa'di AR, Ilahi F, Sheikh SS. The spectrum of breast diseases in Saudi Arab females: a 26-year pathological survey at Dhahran health center. Ann Saudi Med. 1995;15(2): 125-32. [PubMed] [Google Scholar]

3) Adesunkanmi AR, Agbakwuru EA. Benign breast disease at Wesley guild hospital, Ilesha, Nigeria. West Afr J Med. 2001;20(2): 146-51. [PubMed] [Google Scholar]

4) Kim MJ, Kim EK, Park SY, Jung HK, Oh KK, Seok JY. Galactoceles mimicking suspicious solid masses on sonography. J Ultrasound Med. 2006;25(2): 145-51. [PubMed] [Google Scholar]

5) James M, Winkler MD. Galactocele of the breast. Am J Surg. 1964;108(3): 357-60. [PubMed] [Google Scholar]
6) Stevens K, Burrell HC, Evans AJ, Sibbering DM. The ultrasound appearances of galactocoeles. Br J Radiol. 1997;70(831): 239-41. [PubMed] [Google Scholar]
7) Gomez A, Mata JM, Donoso L, Rams A. Galactocele: three distinctive radiographic appearances. Radiology. 1986;158(1): 43-4. [PubMed] [Google Scholar]

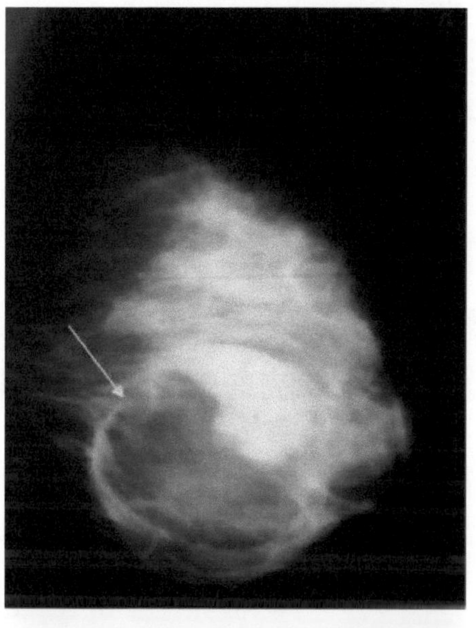

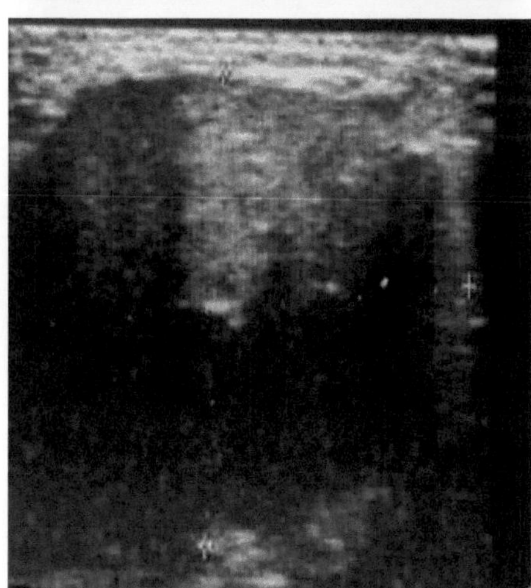

Figure 1. a. Mammography of galactocele: A circumscribed, round mass with circumscribed contours in a double radiolucent tone, associated with fat, while those with a denser content will

be radio-opaque, associated with milk. b. Level I mammary ultrasound: A well-circumscribed, round mass with circumscribed liquid-liquid contours.

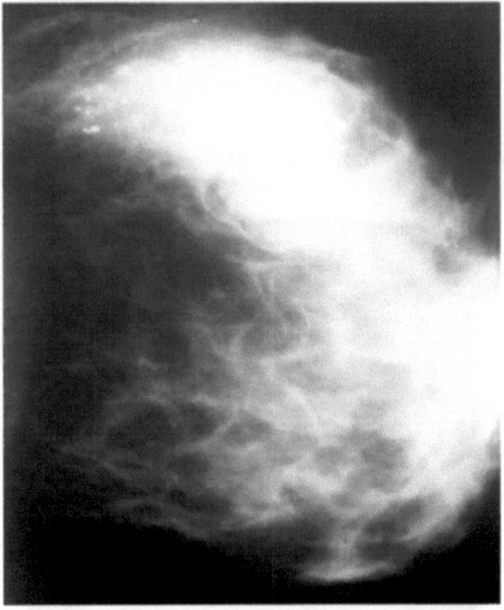

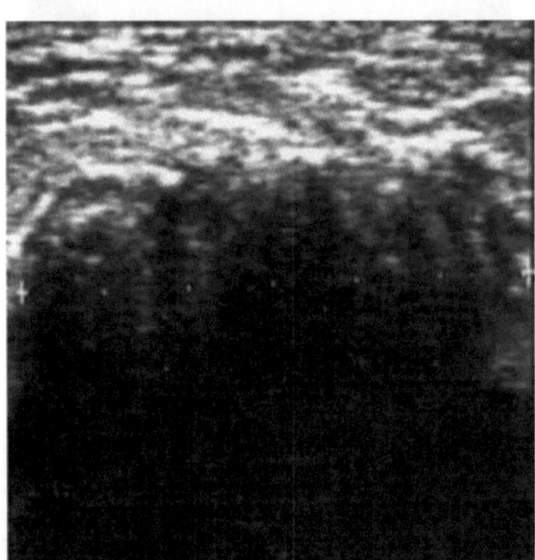

Figure 2, a. Mammogram of galactocele: A well circumscribed, oval mass with circumscribed contours in places, masked in others.

b. Ultrasound mammary well circumscribed mass, round or oval with circumscribed contours containing floating internal echoes.

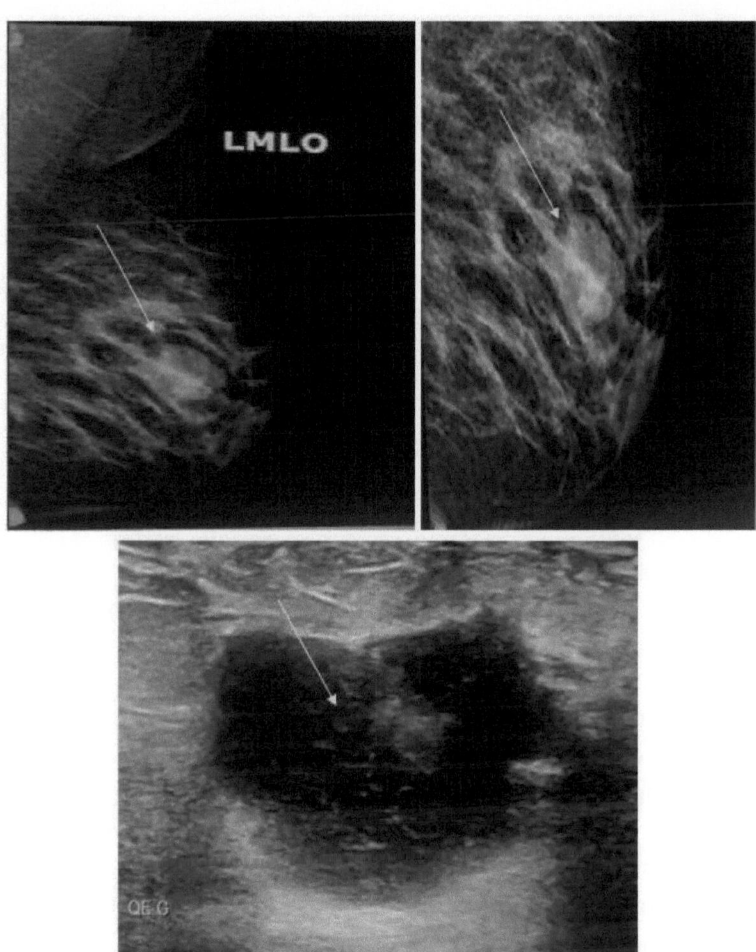

Figure 3, a. Mammogram of galactocele: A well-circumscribed, oval mass with circumscribed contours.

b. Mammary ultrasound of galactocele: lobulated mass, well circumscribed in places, containing floating internal echoes.

VII. Imaging breast lipomas

1. Introduction

Mammary lipomas are benign tumours composed of mature adipose tissue. Although they are generally considered to be benign lesions, imaging plays an important role in their diagnosis and characterisation.

2. Epidemiology

Can occur at any age, including in men.

3. Pathophysiology

Benign tumours composed exclusively of adipose tissue which generally grow slowly and do not tend to infiltrate surrounding tissue.

4. Clinical presentation

Often asymptomatic and discovered incidentally on imaging or palpation. May present as a palpable, soft, mobile, painless mass.

5. Imaging methods

5.1. Mammography

Mammography is often used as the primary imaging modality for assessing breast lipomas. Radiological features of breast lipomas on mammography include:

1) A well-circumscribed mass, oval or round in shape, with smooth circumscribed contours;
2) Low radiological density, related to the lipid content of the lipoma.
3) An absence of significant calcifications, although punctiform calcifications may sometimes be present;
4) Breast lipomas are often located in adipose tissue, at a distance from the glandular parenchyma.

5.2. Ultrasound

Ultrasound is an essential imaging modality for characterising breast lipomas. It is usually hypoechoic with the same echostructure as the subcutaneous fat, crossed by fine trabeculae. Less often, the lipoma is hyperechoic, which Linda explains by a high density of compactly arranged adipocytes, creating multiple interfaces. Sonographic features of breast lipomas include:

1) A well-defined mass with smooth contours;
2) Weak or mixed echogenicity, due to the presence of adipose tissue;
3) Homogeneous ultrasound texture;
4) Mammary lipomas are generally located in the subcutaneous tissue or in the mammary floor.

5.3. MRI (Magnetic Resonance Imaging)

MRI is a sensitive and specific imaging modality used in breast imaging to detect and characterise breast lipomas. MRI features include :

Appearance :

1) A well-defined mass with smooth contours;
2) A hyperintense signal in T1 and suppression of the signal in fat saturation;
3) No enhancement after injection of contrast medium ;
4) Breast lipomas may be located in adipose tissue or close to glandular parenchyma.

6. Conclusion

Imaging plays an essential role in the diagnosis and characterisation of breast lipomas. Breast lipomas are benign adipose lesions with distinct imaging features that facilitate their diagnosis. A thorough understanding of these features enables appropriate management, minimising unnecessary interventions and anxiety for patients.

7. References

1) Journo G, Bataillon G, Benchimol R, Bekhouche A, Dratwa C, Sebbag-Sfez D et al. Hyperechoic breast images: all that glitters is not gold! Insights Imaging 2018; 9: 199-209.

2) American College of Radiology. Illustrated breast imaging reporting and date system (BIRADS), 3rd edn. Reston: American College of Radiology, 2013.

3) Stavros AT, Thickman D, Rapp CI, Denis MA, Parker SH, Sisney GA. Solid breast nodules: use of sonography to distinguish between benign and malignant lesions. Radiology 1995; 196: 123-124.

4) Linda A, Zuiani C, Lorenzon M, Furlan A, Girometti R, Londero V et al. Hyperechoic lesions of the breast: not always benign. AJR 2011; 196: 1219-1224

5) Linda A, Zuiani C, Lorenzon M, Furlan A, Londero V, Machin P et al. The wide spectrum of hyperechoic lesions of the breast. Clin Radiol 2011; 66: 559-565.

6) Fouque O, Kind M, Boulet B, Brisse H, Kemel S, Genah I et al. Diagnostic strategy in the face of a fatty soft tissue tumour in adults. J Imag Diagn Interv 2018; 1: 265- 283.

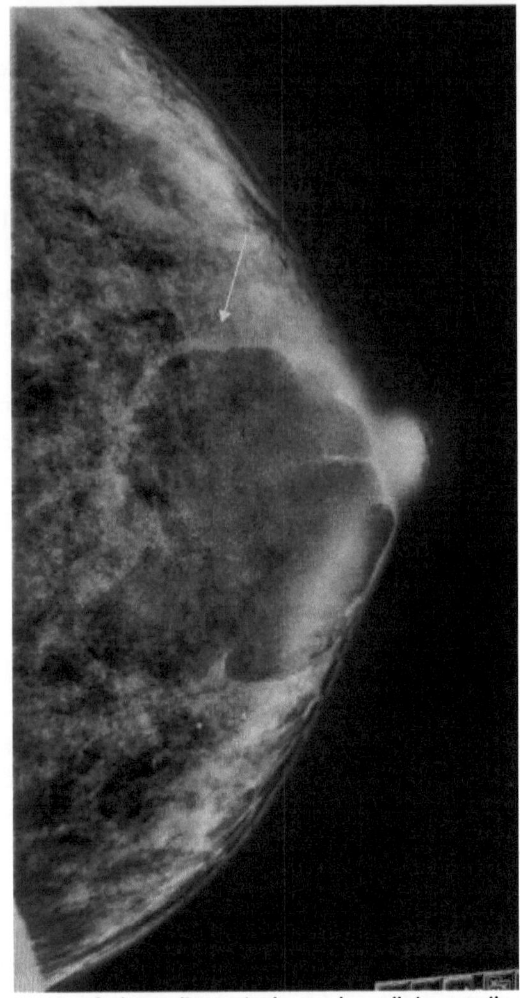

Figure 1: Mammogram of a breast lipoma in the areola: well circumscribed, homogeneous retroareolar clearness, with no microcalcification.

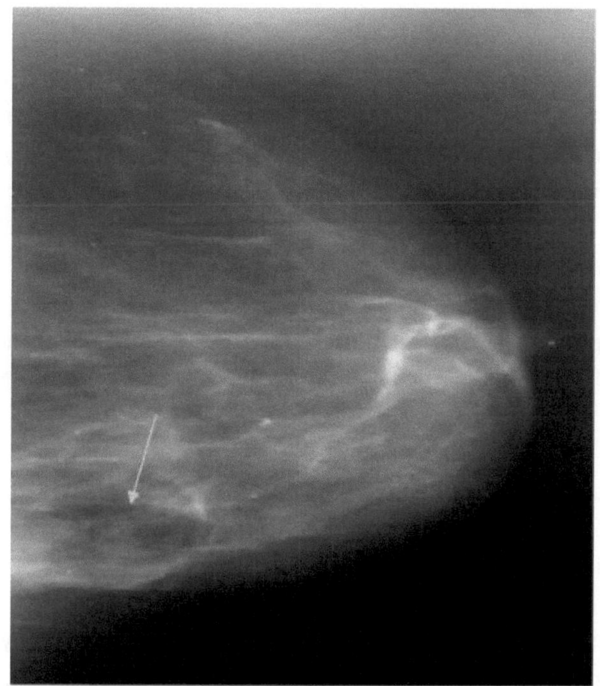

Figure 2. Mammography, front view, a. Radiolucent, well circumscribed, homogeneous clearness of the inner quadrant.

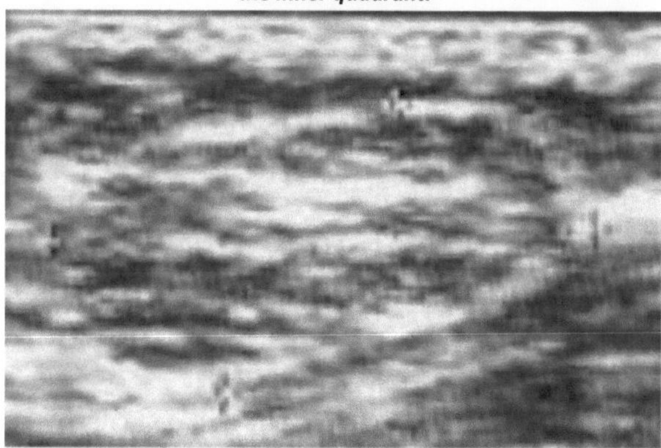

Figure 3: Mammary ultrasound: oval-shaped mass with circumscribed contours, isoechoic, homogeneous.

VIII. Imaging mammary oil cysts

1. Introduction

Breast oil cysts, also known as cystic lip necrosis, are a particular form of benign breast lesion. They often result from trauma or previous surgery, leading to necrosis of fatty tissue and accumulation of lipids inside a cystic cavity. This data sheet is designed to help you assess and characterise breast oil cysts using different imaging techniques.

2. Epidemiology

Oily cysts can occur at any age, but are more frequently diagnosed in middle-aged and older women, particularly those who have undergone breast trauma or surgery.

3. Pathophysiology

Cystic liponecrosis occurs when breast fat tissue is damaged, leading to necrosis and the formation of cavities filled with lipid material and sometimes cellular debris.

4. Clinical presentation

Oily cysts are often asymptomatic and discovered incidentally during an imaging examination. However, they may appear as a palpable, sometimes tender, mass.

5. Imaging methods

5.1. Mammography

> Oily cysts may appear as round or oval lesions with well-defined contours;

> They show a variable radiological density, with areas of radio transparency due to the lipid content;

> Peripheral or intracystic calcifications may occur as a result of scarring or necrosis.

5.2. Ultrasound

> On ultrasound, oily cysts may show variable echogenicity, often with a central anechoic appearance due to the lipid content;

> The walls of the cyst may be thickened and calcified, reflecting an inflammatory or scarring process;

> Posterior acoustic reinforcement may be present, indicating the liquid nature of the contents.

5.3. MRI (Magnetic Resonance Imaging)

> On MRI, oily cysts typically show a hyperintense signal on T1 sequences, characteristic of lipid tissue;

> Suppression of the signal in sequences with fat saturation confirms the presence of lipids.

> Minimal or no enhancement after injection of contrast medium indicates a predominantly cystic and benign nature.

6. Conclusion

Breast oil cysts are benign lesions resulting from the necrosis of fatty tissue. They have distinct imaging features that help to differentiate them from other breast lesions.

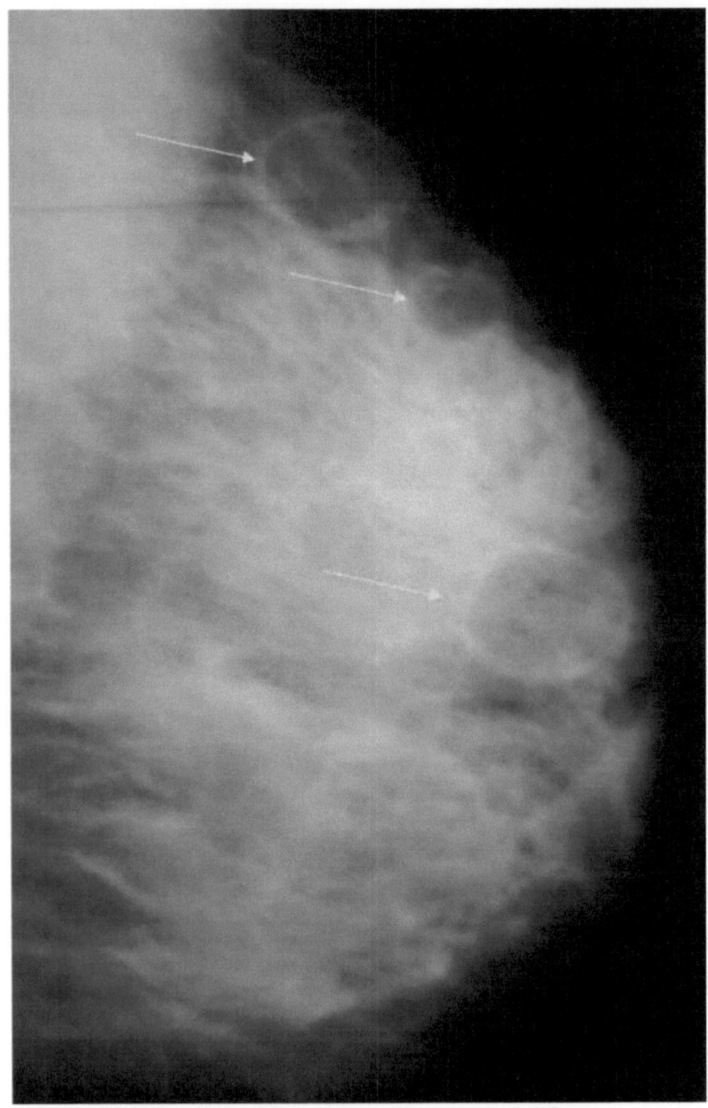

Figure 1. Mammogram. Oily cyst. Rounded, circumscribed, scattered clefts.

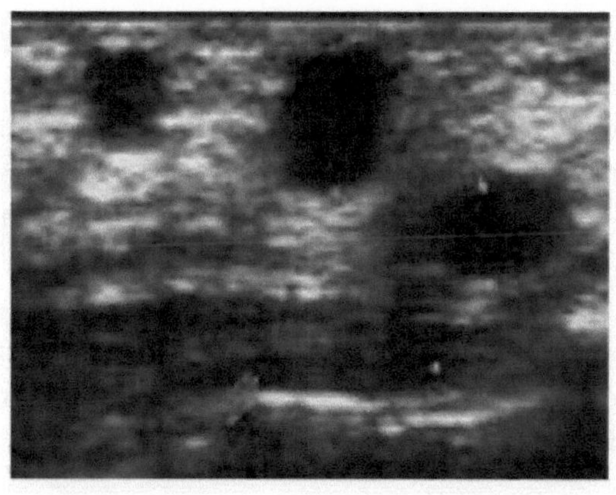

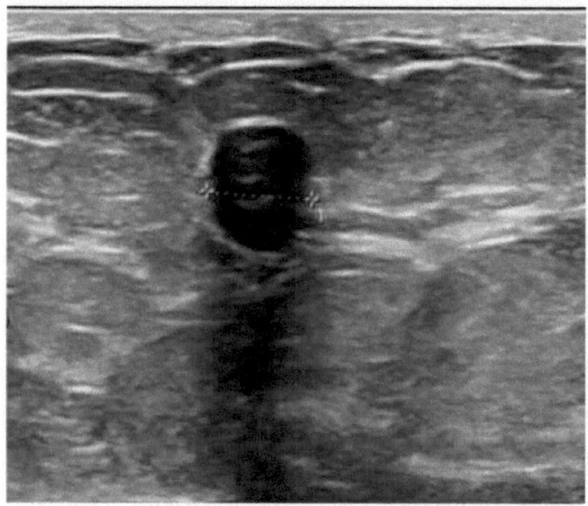

Figure 2. Breast ultrasound. Oily cyst. Cysts, rounded, anechoic within fatty tissue, circumscribed, scattered.

IX. Imaging intramammary lymph nodes

1. Introduction

Intramammary lymph nodes are normal lymphatic structures present in breast tissue. Although they are generally benign, their identification and characterisation are important to exclude associated malignant pathologies. They are class BI. RADS 2 of the ACR.

2. Etiology

Intramammary nodes are lymph nodes located within the breast tissue. They may become more apparent or palpable as a result of hormonal changes, infections, inflammatory processes or reactions to trauma.

3. Imaging methods

3.1. Mammography

Intramammary nodes appear as round or oval masses with a radiolucent centre or notch, the dense component of which has circumscribed contours, imitating a "target" or "halo". They are generally located in the superior-external region of the breast opposite a vascular axis. Mammography can detect the presence of intra-breast nodes, but may require other imaging modalities for a complete characterisation.

3.2. Mammary ultrasound

The intra-mammary ganglion has a central hypoechoic appearance (the ganglion sinus) surrounded by a regular echogenic cortex measuring less than 3 mm. The shape is generally oval, kidney-shaped and oriented parallel to the skin.

Ultrasound is highly effective in characterising intramammary nodes, demonstrating their internal structure and enabling benign nodes to be distinguished from suspicious solid lesions.

3.3. Magnetic Resonance Imaging (MRI) of the breast

Intramammary nodes may show maximum enhancement after injection of gadolinium, with a Wachs out in T1 and T2.

MRI is used in cases where mammography and ultrasound are not sufficient to rule out malignant pathology, offering a detailed assessment of lymph node morphology and vascularisation.

4. Differential diagnosis

> Lymph node metastases ;

> Fibroadenomas ;

> Complex cysts.

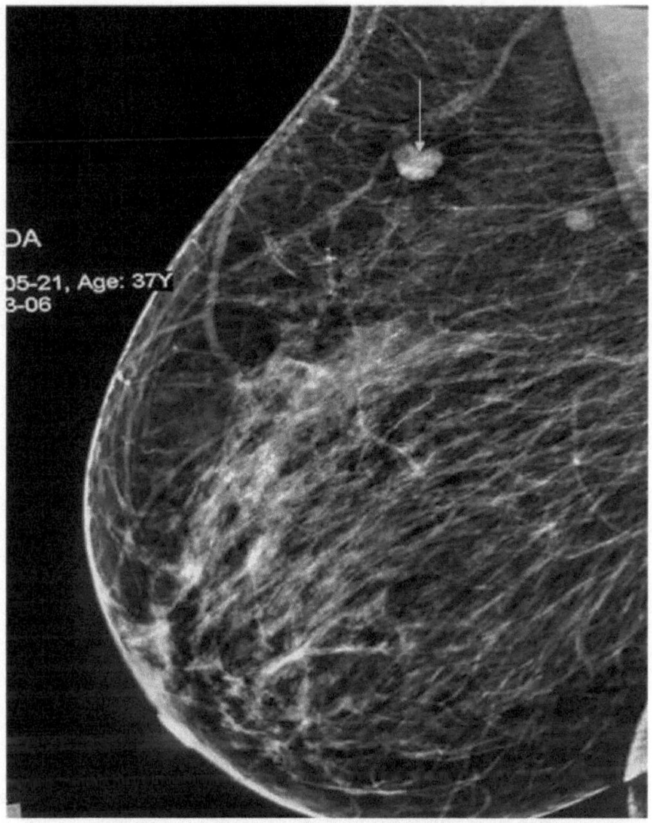

Figure 1. right external oblique mammogram. Intra-breast node with peripheral cortical notch in the upper quadrant, opposite a vascular axis (arrow).

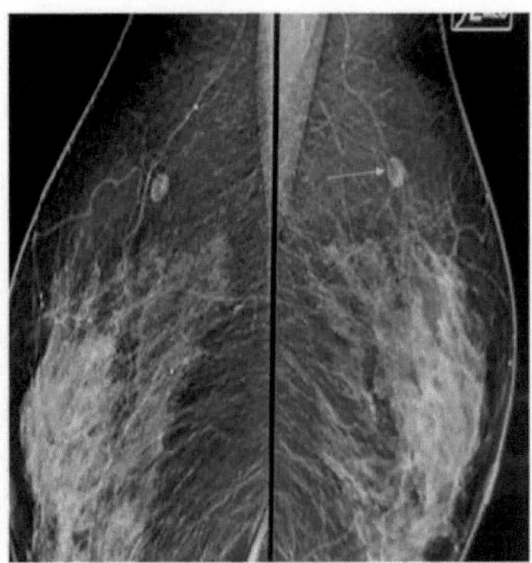

Figure 2: Bilateral mammogram with external oblique views. Intra mammary nodes, with central clearness, located in the upper quadrant, opposite a vascular axis. (arrow)

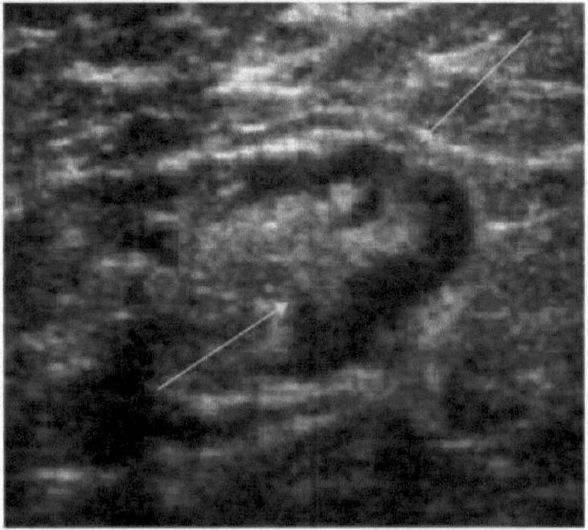

Figure 3: Mammary ultrasound. Intra mammary node, oval with hypoechoic cortex, thin and regular, and a central fatty hilum (arrow).

X. Imaging Breast Fibroadenomas

1. Introduction

Fibroadenomas are one of the most common benign breast tumours, especially in young women. Although they are generally benign, their accurate assessment by imaging is important in distinguishing fibroadenomas from other breast lesions, particularly those of a malignant nature.

2. Etiology

Fibroadenomas are of lobular origin with two epithelial and connective contingents. The risk of degeneration is very low (1/10,000).

Fibroadenomas are influenced by hormones, particularly restrogens, and are therefore more common in young women of childbearing age. They can vary in size, number and appearance over time, particularly during pregnancy and breast-feeding. It can be complex when associated with cysts, sclerosing adenoses, calcifications and apocrine and papillary changes.

3. Imaging methods

3.1. Mammography

Fibroadenomas appear as well circumscribed, oval or round masses, sometimes lobulated with or without coarse calcifications. They are generally isolated from the surrounding glandular tissue.

Mammography is important for detecting and locating fibroadenomas, as well as looking for changes such as the presence of microcalcifications associated with degeneration, which remains exceptional. Ultrasound is often necessary for a more precise characterisation.

With age, fibroadenomas tend to regress and calcify, with typical calcifications being "popcorn" or "coral-shaped".

3.2. Mammary ultrasound

Fibroadenomas appear as solid, well circumscribed, hypoechoic, homogeneous lesions with an oval shape and smooth margins, with a long axis parallel to the cutaneous plane, showing posterior enhancement. Posterior acoustic attenuation is rare.

Ultrasound provides a detailed study of the internal echostructure of the fibroadenoma, making it easier to distinguish between benign and suspicious lesions and guide interventional imaging procedures.

3.3. Magnetic Resonance Imaging (MRI) of the breast

On MRI, fibroadenomas generally show an oval mass with circumscribed iso- or hypointense contours in T1 and a frank T2 hypersignal that varies according to

the tissue content. epithelial component (favouring hypersignal) compared with the fibrous component (favouring hyposignal).
Bulkheads can be detected on T2 (windowing must be optimal) or on native contrast-negative injected sequences. The absence of enhancement of the septa in fibroadenomas is characteristic.
The dynamic haemodynamic behaviour of a fibroadenoma is typically that of a benign tumour, i.e. slow, centrifugal, homogeneous and progressive with a secondary plateau.
With age, fibroadenomas tend to regress and calcify, with typical calcifications being "popcorn" or "coral-shaped".

4. Differential diagnosis

- Cysts with echogenic content ;
- Phyllodes tumours ;
- Certain triple-negative breast cancers.

5. Care and Support

Small asymptomatic fibroadenomas can simply be monitored for any changes in size or characteristics. They are classified as ACR BI-RADS 3.
A biopsy may be recommended for atypical fibroadenomas, those that change rapidly, or if the distinction with a malignant lesion cannot be established. Surgery is considered for large, symptomatic fibroadenomas, or those that give the patient cause for concern.

6. References

1) Cecilia JI, Miller A, Balassanian R, Mukhtar RA. Early onset, multiple, bilateral fibroadenomas of the breast: a case report. BMC Women's Health. 2021, 21: 170

2) Amshel CE, Sibley E. Multiple unilateral fibroadenomas. The breast journal. 2001;7(3): 189-91.

3) Vinod A, Ashok KR, Gajendra SR, Shashi R. MultipleFibroadenomas in Bilateral Breasts of A 20-Year-old Woman - A Rare Case Report. AJCRS. 2020;3(1): 19-22.

4) Michelle L, Hooman TS. Breast fibroadenomas in adolescents: current perspectives. Adolescent Health, Medicine and Therapeutics 2015: 6 159-163.

5) CAMARA O, EGBE A, KOCH I, HERRMANN J, GAJDA M, BALTZER P, RUNNEBAUM IB. Surgical Management of Multiple Bilateral Fibroadenomaof the Breast: The Ribeiro Technique Modified by Rezai. ANTICANCER RESEARCH. 2009, 29: 28232826

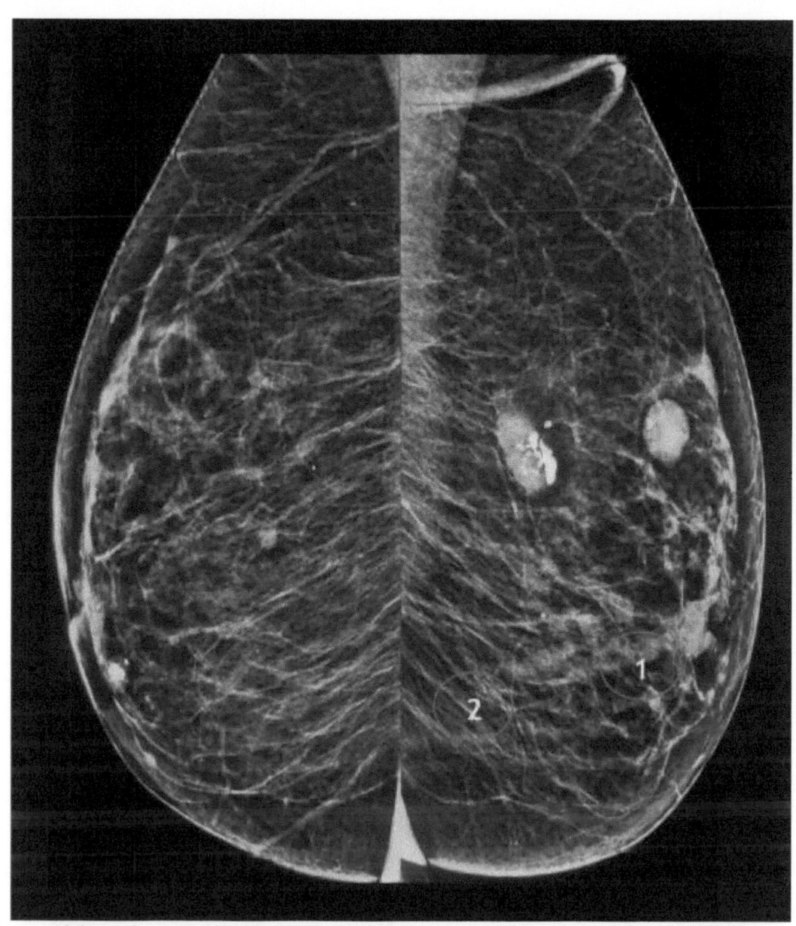

Figure 1. bilateral mammograms, external oblique views. Left breast masses, oval in shape, with circumscribed contours, homogeneous (1), heterogeneous, with coralliform calcifications (2).

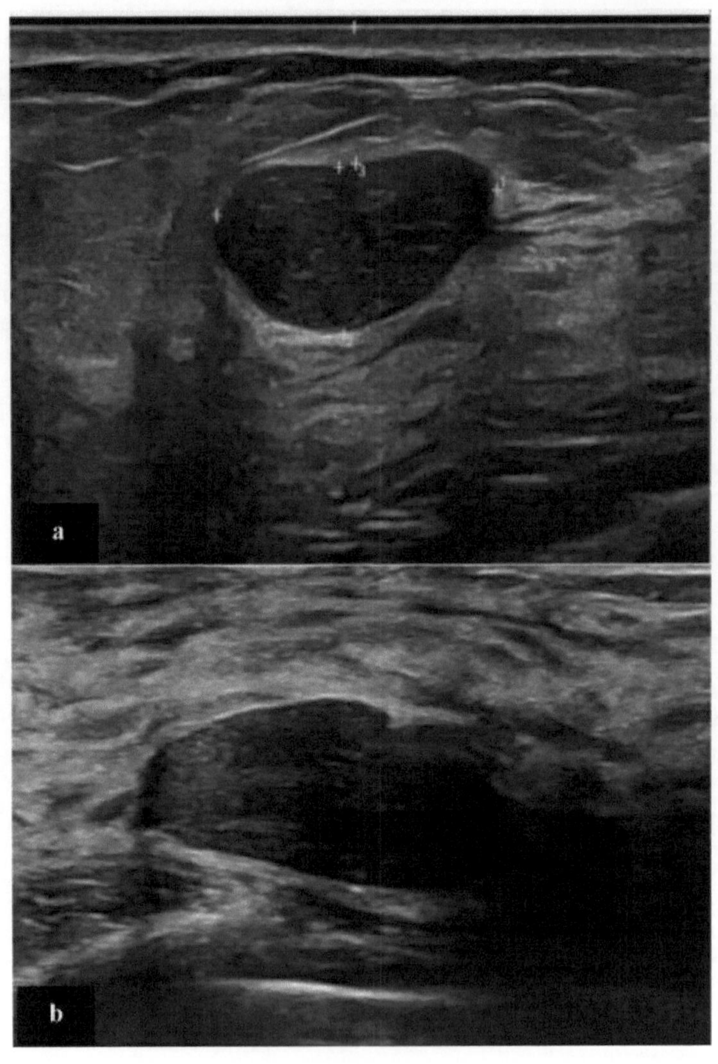
a
b

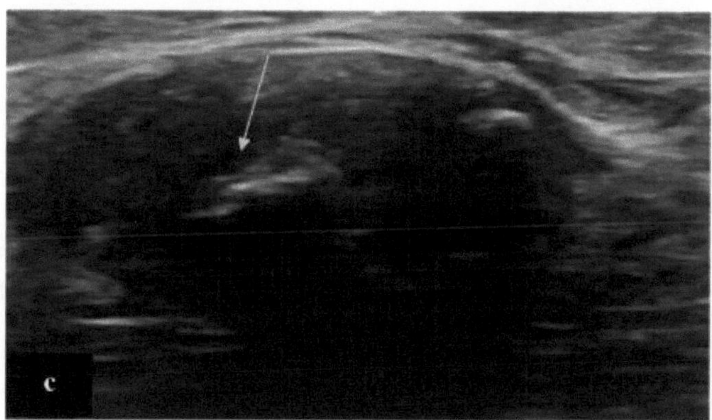

Figure 2. Breast ultrasound. Breast masses (a) oval, hypoechoic, homogeneous, with long axis parallel to the skin planes, with circumscribed contours, (b) lobulated, hypoechoic, homogeneous, with long axis parallel to the skin planes, with circumscribed contours, (c) oval, with circumscribed contours, hypoechoic, heterogeneous due to the presence of calcifications within it, with axis parallel to the skin planes.

CHAPTER 2

XI. Giant juvenile breast adenofibroma

1. Introduction

Juvenile giant fibroadenoma is a rare benign breast disease. It accounts for 2 to 4% of breast fibroadenomas. Giant fibroadenoma is a particular form of fibroadenoma, defined simply by a size greater than 5 cm in diameter. Its pathophysiological mechanism is poorly understood, and it is thought to be the result of an inappropriate local response to oestrogen stimulation.

2. Imaging

2.1. Mammography

Mammography is often used as a second imaging modality to assess giant juvenile breast adenofibromas. Radiological features of these lesions on mammography include:

A limited mass, often round or oval in shape, with circumscribed contours. Variable density, usually fibroglandular.

2.2. Ultrasound

Ultrasonography of the breast is an essential, first-line imaging modality in young women, enabling giant juvenile breast adenofibromas to be characterised. The ultrasound features of these lesions include:

The presence of patches of heterogeneous echo-structure with anechoic cystic areas suggests the existence of haemorrhagic or necrotic areas. There are no pathognomonic signs, but the diagnosis of a phyllodes tumour may be suggested by the presence of lobulations and indistinct contours, associated with cystic areas. On Doppler, it may be avascular, with minimal internal vascularity in 67% of cases and central vessels in 33%.

2.3. MRI (Magnetic Resonance Imaging)

Breast MRI can be used to assess giant juvenile breast adenofibromas in specific cases. MRI features include:

A well-limited mass, often oval or lobulated in shape and circumscribed. A variable signal depending on the tissue composition of the lesion, with a fibrous stromal component and areas of variable signal intensity. The giant juvenile mammary adenofibromas can be located in any part of the breast. This fibro-epithelial tumour shares many histological similarities with the low-grade phyllodes tumour. Both are fibro-epithelial tumours with high stromal cellularity.

However, unlike the phyllodes tumour, this form cellular adenofibroma does not recur and is not malignant in adolescents.

There is a real diagnostic difficulty between giant fibroadenoma and grade I phyllodes tumour. Giant adenofibromas are differentiated from phyllodes by the presence of a true capsule and a more harmonious distribution of stroma and epithelium.

3. Conclusion

Imaging plays an essential role in the evaluation of giant juvenile breast adenofibromas. Mammography, ultrasound and, in some cases, breast MRI are complementary modalities that can be used to characterise these lesions and differentiate them from other malignant or benign lesions. Accurate radiological assessment and appropriate characterisation can confirm the diagnosis of giant juvenile breast adenofibroma and guide clinical management.

4. References

1) Morris A., Shaffer K. Recurrent bilateral giant fibradenomas of the breasts. Radiolog. Case Reports 2007,2(3): 1-5.

2) Chang DS, McGrath MH. Management of benign tumors of the adolescent breast. Plast. Reconstr. Surg. July 2007;120(1): 13e-19e.

3) . Hawary M. B., Cardoso E., Mahmud S., Hassanain J. Giant breast tumors. Ann. Saud. Med. 1999,19(2): 174- 176

4) Marie Roux. Giant fibroadenoma in adolescents and hormonal influence: analysis a series of 90 cases (Thesis 2013).

5) Dalia Gobbi,Patrizia Dall'Igna,RitaAlaggio, DonatoNitti, Giovanni Cecchetto: Giantfibroadenoma of the breast in the adolscents : report of 2 cases: Received 26 August 2008;Revised 10 November 2008,accepted 10 November 2008

6) CABARET V., DELOBELLE-DEROIDE A., VILAIN M. O. Les tumeurs phyllodes. Arch AnatCytol Pathol. 1985; 43(1-2): 59-72.

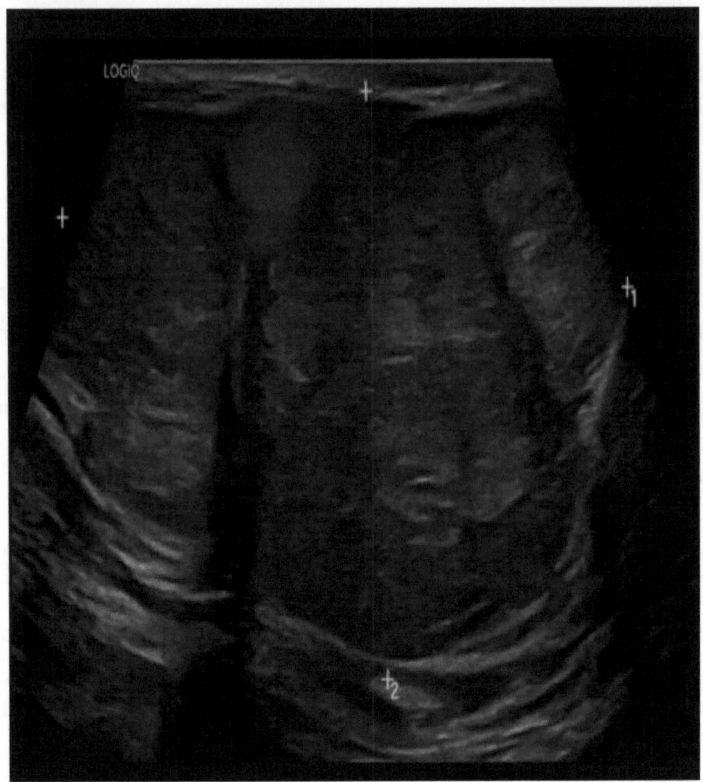

Figure 1, Roughly oval mass with circumscribed contours in some areas, lobulated in others, hypoechoic, heterogeneous, cystic in some areas, ACR BI-RADS 4 classification.

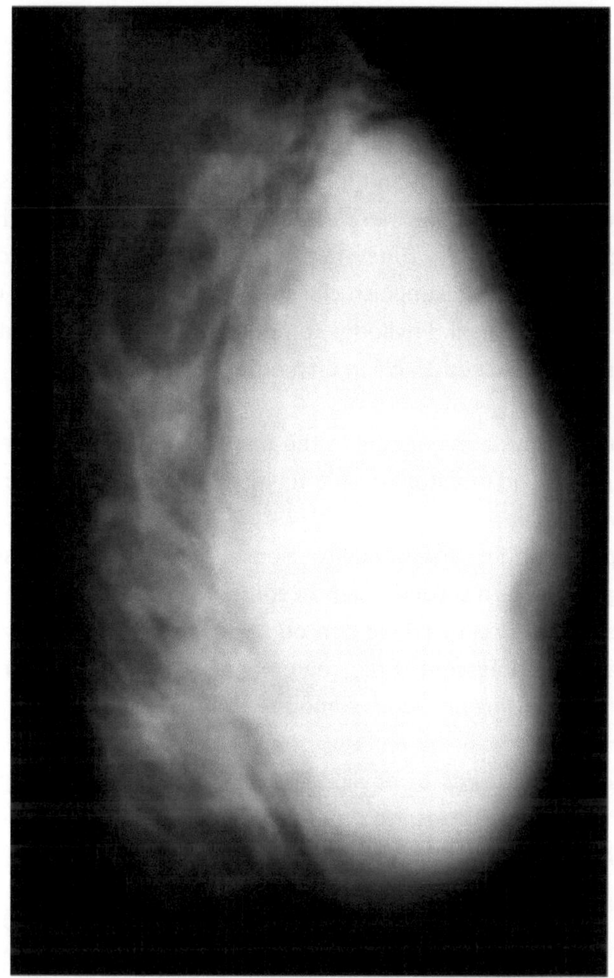

Figure 2, A roughly oval-shaped mass, with circumscribed contours in places, masked by screening in others, homogeneous without microcalcifications within it, classified as ACR BI-RADS 4a.

XII. Phyllodes tumour

1. Introduction

The phyllodes tumour is a rare fibroepithelial tumour of the breast, characterised by rapid growth and local invasiveness. Although this tumour is more common in adult women, cases in adolescent girls have been documented. Clinically, these tumours often present as a firm, rapidly growing nodule that is difficult to distinguish clinically from adenofibromas, particularly when the lesions are small. Phyllodes tumours can reach significant sizes, and in 15% of cases they exceed 15 cm in diameter.

2. Imaging methods

Medical imaging plays a major role in the management of phyllodes tumours, enabling diagnosis and monitoring, characterisation and therapeutic planning.

2.1. Mammography

Mammography is an imaging modality used to assess breast masses, even in adolescent girls, but as a second-line procedure. Mammography can show well-limited masses with circumscribed contours. However, because of the density of the breast in adolescent girls, mammography may have limitations in accurately characterising phyllodes tumours.

2.2. Ultrasound

Typical ultrasound features of phyllodes tumours include a solid, hypoechoic mass with cystic areas. Ultrasound enabled us to visualise the lesion in detail and establish a first level of suspicion of a phyllodes tumour.

2.3. MRI (Magnetic Resonance Imaging)

For a more in-depth characterisation of the lesion, MRI is a powerful imaging modality that provides additional information on the vascularisation, size and extension of breast lesions.

However, MRI is generally only performed if there is a strong suspicion of malignancy, as there is no specific semiology that clearly distinguishes benign from malignant phyllodes tumours.

General characteristics

Phyllodes tumours generally present as masses that may be well-defined or have irregular contours, depending on whether they are benign or malignant. On T1-weighted sequences, phyllodes may show an isointense or slightly hyperintense signal compared with the surrounding mammary glandular tissue. On T2-weighted sequences, they may show a heterogeneous signal, with hyperintense areas due to the presence of cystic or haemorrhagic components, or myxoid degeneration. After injection of gadolinium, phyllodes tumours generally show enhancement. Benign tumours tend to have a homogeneous and progressive enhancement, often plateau-like, similar to that of fibroadenomas.

Malignant or high-grade tumours may show more heterogeneous and rapid enhancement with areas of wash-out, indicating irregular vascularisation and potentially greater aggressiveness.

Cystic remodelling and areas of necrosis may be associated with a higher degree of malignancy.

It is important to note that, although MRI can provide valuable clues as to the nature of the tumour, the formal distinction between benign, borderline and malignant phyllodes tumours is based on histological examination.

In summary, MRI is a valuable tool for assessing the local extension of phyllodes tumours, guiding surgical planning, and in some cases, helping to assess the potential for malignancy. However, MRI features are not specific and must be interpreted in the overall clinical context, in conjunction with histological findings for an accurate assessment.

Ultrasound-guided microbiopsies remain essential for accurate preoperative histological diagnosis.

3. Conclusion

The most common curative treatment for a phyllodes tumour wide surgical excision with margins of more than 1 cm. Apart from surgery, there is no definitive cure for phyllodes tumours, as neither chemotherapy nor radiotherapy has proven effective. However, radiation treatment after breast-conserving surgery with negative margins can significantly reduce the rate local recurrence for borderline and malignant tumours.

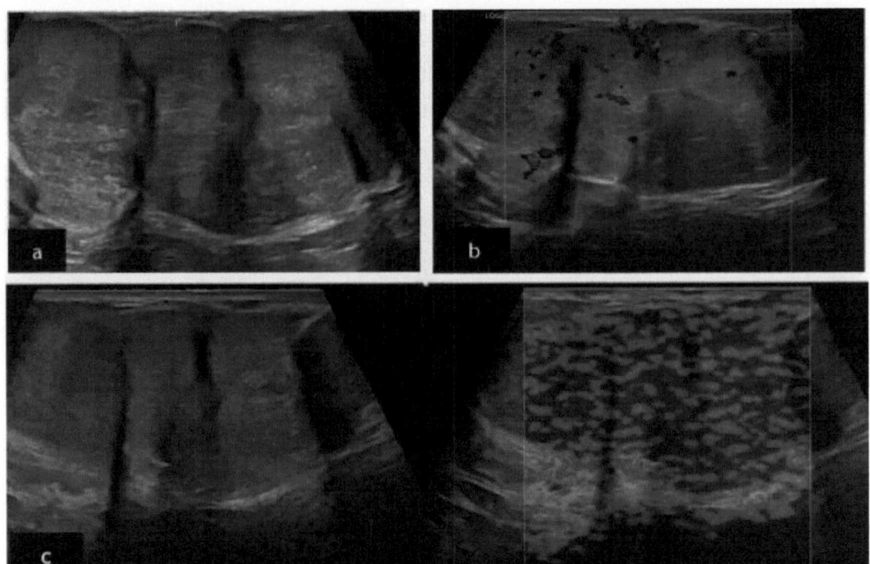

Figure 1. a. B-mode mammary ultrasound: lobulated mass with circumscribed contours, heterogeneous due to the presence of one cystic mass. b. Vascularised on Doppler c, Intermediate consistency on elastography.

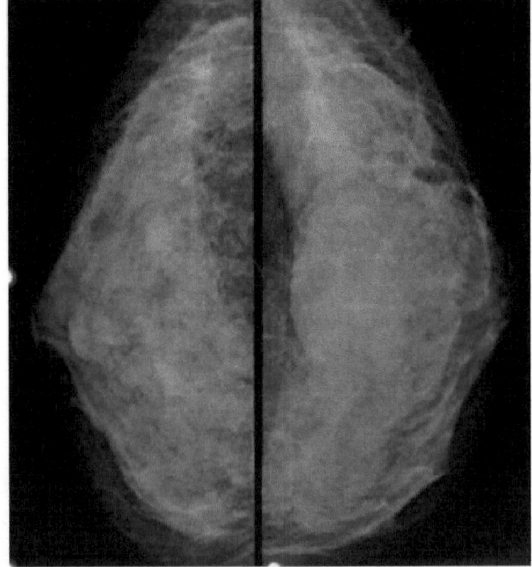

Figure 2: Bilateral mammogram, face-on views: left mass, roughly lobulated, homogeneous, with circumscribed contours in places, masks in other places in relation to a grade 1 phyllodes.

4. References

1) Abdulcadir D, Nori J, Meattini I, Giannotti E, Boeri C, Vanzi E, et al. Phyllodes tumours of the breast diagnosed as B3 category on image-guided 14-gauge

core biopsy: analysis of 51 cases from a single institution and review of the literature. Eur J Surg Oncol 2014;40: 859-64. 1028 S. Bendifallah, G. Canlorbe

2) Spitaleri G, Toesca A, Botteri E, Bottiglieri L, Rotmensz N, Boselli S, et al. Breast phyllodes tumor: a review of literature and a single center retrospective series analysis. Crit Rev Oncol Hematol 2013;88: 427-36.

3) Bennett IC, Khan A, De Freitas R, Chaudary MA, Millis RR. Phyllodes tumours: a clinicopathological review of 30 cases. Aust N Z J Surg 1992;62: 628-33.

4) Liberman L, Bonaccio E, Hamele-Bena D, et al. Benign and malignant phyllodes tumors: mammographic and sonographic findings. Radiology 1996; 198: 121-4.

5) Yabuuchi H, Soeda H, Matsuo Y, et al. Phyllodes tumor of the breast. Correlation between MR findings and histologic grade. Radiology 2006; 241 : 7.

6) Kim S, Kim J-Y, Kim DH, Jung WH, Koo JS. Analysis of phyllodes tumor recurrence according to the histologic grade. Breast Cancer Res Treat 2013;141: 353-63

XIII. Imaging mammary hamartomas

1. Introduction

Hamartomas are defined as rare benign tumours. They represent approximately 0.7% of all benign mammary masses. They are lesions made up of varying proportions of the normal histological constituents of the parenchyma of the organ in which they develop. They can occur in several organs such as the lung, skin and breast.

Clinically, mammary hamartoma is generally asymptomatic, but can manifest itself, as in the case of our patient, as a firm, mobile tissue nodule.

2. Imaging

The diagnosis is made using standard mammography and breast ultrasound imaging.

2.1. Mammography

Mammography is often used as the primary imaging modality for assessing breast hamartomas. In mammography, the diagnosis is almost pathognomonic, revealing a round, oval breast mass with circumscribed contours surrounded by a halo, a thin, clear radiolucent border corresponding to the pseudocapsule, of variable density, within which are juxtaposed fatty spots and more or less dense opacities producing the typical "sausage slice" appearance.

A "breast in the breast" appearance and the appearance of a double component: radiolucent, fatty and dense due to the presence of fibro-glandular tissue are also described, depending on the make-up of the breast tissue (fat, gland, fibrous tissue) within the mass.

Microcalcifications or dystrophic calcifications are rarely seen within a hamartoma.

2.2. Ultrasound

Ultrasound reveals a mass with circumscribed contours, oval in shape. Most often, there is no posterior enhancement or attenuation cone.

This mass is heterogeneous, with isoechoic areas of fat and hyperechoic areas like normal glandular tissue. It may be the site of a galactocele or simple cyst.

2.3. MRI (Magnetic Resonance Imaging)

Breast MRI is not indicated unless there are signs of malignancy. MRI reveals a well-limited, encapsulated mass in T1 hyposignal, heterogeneous due to the presence of breast tissue, enhancing after injection of contrast medium with an unenhanced peripheral border, suggesting a hamartoma. The appearance is often described as a "breast within a breast", with fat and matrix tissue to a greater or lesser extent.

From an anatomopathological point of view, the Hamartoma is made up of variable numbers of lobules scattered in no particular order, cysts, sometimes with apocrine metaplasia, and connective tissue. This connective tissue is dense, fibrous and sometimes hyaline, forming an annular arrangement around the acini.

The hamartoma follows the evolution of normal mammary parenchyma and undergoes physiological variations as with mammary tissue. With age, normal mammary tissue involutes, which can make the harmatoma much more visible.

The hamartoma of the breast does not degenerate but, due to the presence of normal breast tissue, the development of cancer within the hamartoma is possible. The elements for suspecting cancer are the same as in the breast. 16 cases typical hamartomas have been published in the literature.

3. Action to be taken (CAT)

Although benign, the presence of fibroglandular tissue within the hamartoma makes it possible for a carcinoma to develop. Differential diagnoses include liposarcoma, Cowden's disease, lipoma and fibroadenoma.

4. Treatment

Regular follow-up is recommended to monitor any changes. Surgical may be considered in cases of rapid growth or symptomsexcisionassociated .

5. Conclusion

A breast hamartoma is a volume of histologically normal breast tissue that is circumscribed and therefore often enucleable. The diagnosis of breast hamartoma is easy in its typical form. Mammography alone is sufficient to confirm the diagnosis, avoiding the need for biopsy or systematic surgical removal. Surgical removal should only be considered in cases of discomfort or breast deformity. Breast hamartomas are rarely associated with malignant tumours.

6. References

1) Villeta A, Sáenz D, Ramia JM, Sánchez D, Morales C, Alcalde J, et al. Hamartoma de mama. A propósito de un nuevo caso. Rev Senol Patol Mam 1993;6: 145-9.

2) Yeu YM, Kong JH, Cheung F, Chong SF. Mammary hamartoma: is clinical diagnosis possible? J R Coll Surg Edinb 1997;42: 279-80.

3) . Linell F, Ostberg G, Soderstrom J, Andersson I, Hildell J, Ljungqvist U. Breast hamartomas. An important entity in mammary pathology. Virchows Arch A Pathol Anat Histol 1979;383: 253-64.

4) Travade A, Dauplat J, Fonk Y. Mammary hamartomas. Mammographic and histological aspects. A propos de 5 observations. Rev Fr Gynécol Obstet 1986;81: 37-40.

5) . Jones MW, Norris HJ, Wargotz ES. Hamartoma of the breast. A review. Surgery, Gynecol Obstet 1991;173: 54-6.

6) Blomqvist L, Malm M, Fernstad R. Hamartoma of the breast: surgical treatment and reconstruction. Case report. Scand J Plast Reconstr Surg Hand Surg 1997;31: 365-9. 18. Dworak O, Reck T, Greskotter KR, Kocherling F. Hamartoma of an ectopic breast arising in the inguinal region. Histopathology 1994;24: 169-71

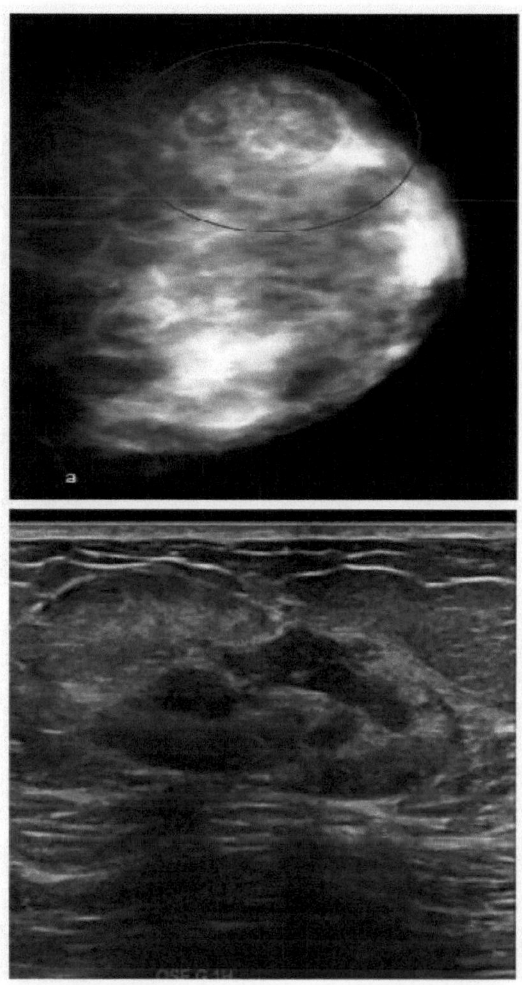

Figure 1a: Mammogram (craniocaudal view): typical mammographic appearance of a mammary hamartoma: oval mass with circumscribed contours and fat density, classified as a hamartoma.
BIRADS2
1b: Breast ultrasound: ultrasound appearance a breast mass: oval mass with circumscribed contours of hypoechoic echostructure, classified BI-RADS 2.

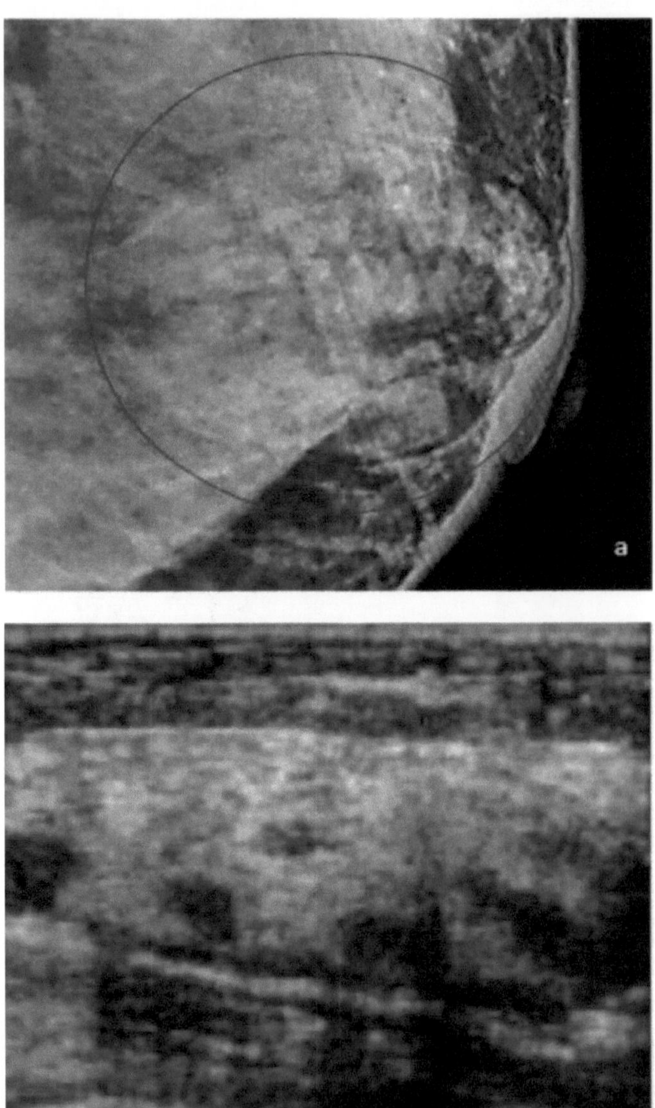

Figure 2a: Mammogram (craniocaudal incidence): typical mammographic appearance of a mammary hamartoma: rounded mass with circumscribed contours of predominantly conjunctival density surrounded by a peripheral halos, classified as BI-RADS 2.

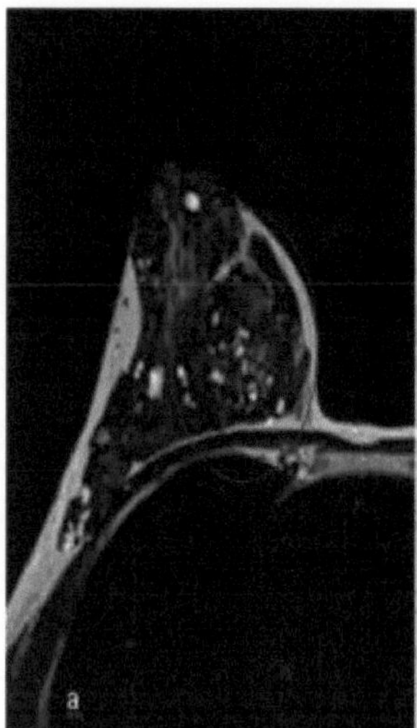

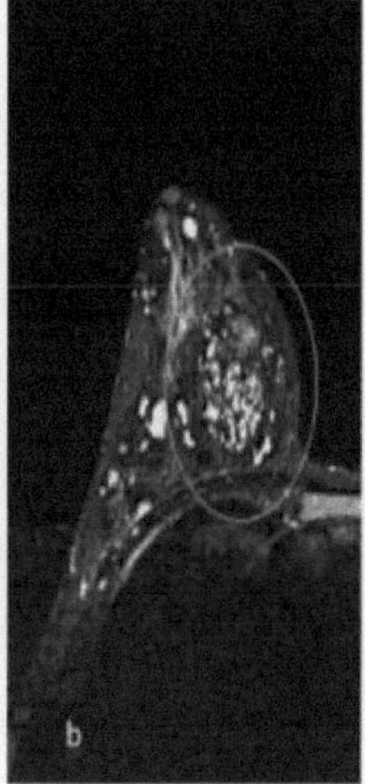

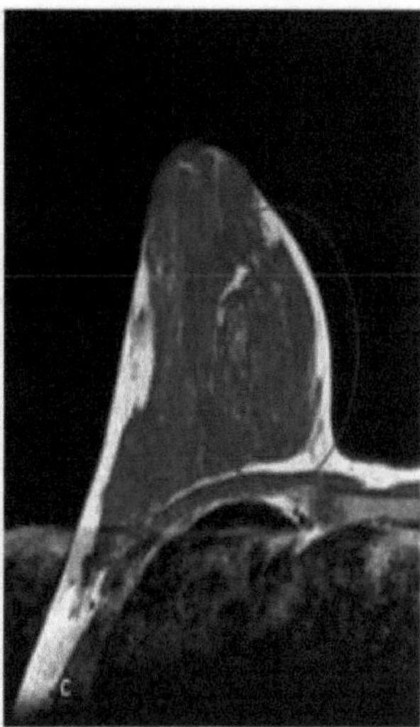

Figure 4: Breast MRI

> *a: T2-weighted axial scan: well-limited mass in the right breast isosignal to the rest of the breast.*

> *b: Axial T1 fat sat: well limited mass of the right breast in hyposignal, heterogeneous. containing microcysts.*

> *c: T1-weighted axial sequence: well-limited mass in the right breast isosignal to the rest of the breast.*

XIV. Radial scar or Aschoff Proliferative Centre (APC)

1. Introduction

Radial scarring, also known as Aschoff's proliferative centre (APC), is a benign breast lesion characterised by a sclerosing proliferation around a ductal centre. It corresponds to a fibrous proliferation surrounding the ductal structures. From a prognostic point of view, these lesions are similar to so-called "complex sclerosing" lesions. It is often associated with proliferating breast lesions and appears to increase the risk of cancer only moderately.

It can sometimes simulate a malignant lesion on imaging due to its spiculated appearance. Accurate distinction on imaging is crucial to avoid unnecessary biopsies and to guide appropriate management.

2. Etiology

The exact causes of radial scarring are not well understood. It is often discovered incidentally imaging examinations or biopsies carried out for other indications. There is no direct link with specific risk factors for breast cancer.

3. Imaging methods

3.1. Mammography

It takes the form of a suspicious mammographic image, usually spiculated with a clear centre and usually without any clinical manifestations.

> The typical appearance is a lesion with radiating spicules starting a less dense centre. Calcifications may be present but are not specific. It most often appears as an irregular mass associated with intra-lobular microcalcifications that look suspicious on mammography;

> Can be difficult to distinguish from invasive carcinoma, often requiring further investigation.

3.2. Mammary ultrasound

> Reveals a hypoechoic lesion with a radial architecture or areas of more echogenic. The contours are irregular due to fibrotic retraction;

> Elastography is used to assess the consistency of the lesion and its relationship with neighbouring structures, helping to differentiate radial scarring from cancers.

3.3. Magnetic Resonance Imaging (MRI) of the breast

> Shows moderate to intense enhancement after injection of gadolinium, with radial architecture. Contrast kinetics can help differentiate radial scarring

from malignant lesions;

> Recommended when the results of mammography and ultrasound are ambiguous or to assess the extent of the lesion.

4. Differential diagnosis

> Carcinoma of the breast, in particular lobular carcinoma or ductal carcinoma in situ ;

> Other forms of mammary sclerosis.

5. Care and Support

> **Biopsy:** A biopsy guided by ultrasound or mammography may be necessary to obtain a definitive diagnosis, particularly in the presence of atypical features or if the distinction with a malignant lesion is not clear;

> **Monitoring:** Benign radial scars without atypia can be monitored regularly, thus avoiding unnecessary surgery;

> **Surgery:** Percutaneous sampling, even macrobiopsy [16], is not sufficiently exhaustive to obviate the need for surgical excision to allow complete histological control. Removal of these lesions therefore remains essential at present.

6. Conclusion

Radial scarring is a benign entity that can mimic a malignant lesion on imaging. Precise characterisation using different imaging modalities is essential to guide appropriate management and avoid over-treatment. Biopsy remains the definitive diagnostic tool, but the approach must be individualised according to radiological features, clinical history and patient preferences.

7. References

1) Sanders ME, Page DL, Simpson JF et al. Interdependence of radial scar and proliferative disease with respect to invasive breast carcinoma risk in patients with benign breast biopsies. Cancer 2006;106(7): 1453-61.

2) PattersonJA, ScottM,AndersonN,Kirk SJ. Radialscar,complex sclerosing lesionandrisk ofbreast cancer. Analysis of 175 cases in Northern Ireland. EurJ Surg Oncol 2004;30(10): 1065-8.

3) Farshid G, Rush G. Assessment of 142 stellate lesions with imaging features suggestive of radial scar discovered during population-based screening for breastcancer. AmJ Surg Pathol 2004;28(12): 1626-31.

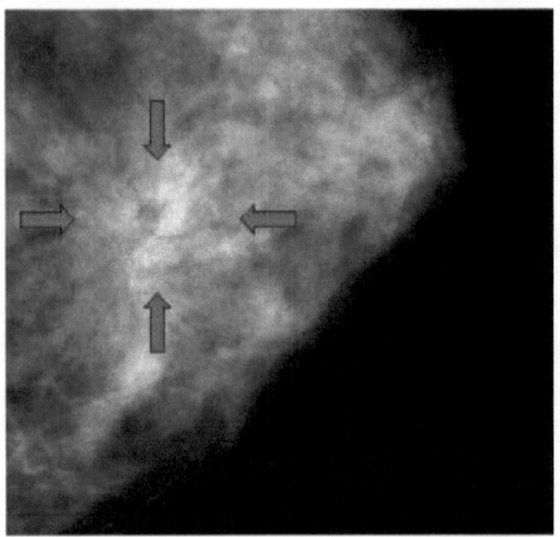

Figure 1: Mammography; Speculated shape and contour mass with dense centre

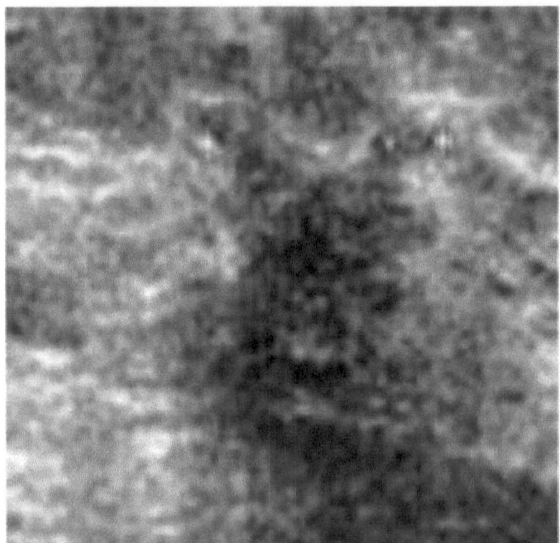

Figure 2. Ultrasound; Hypoechoic, attenuating mass with speculated shape and contours

XV. Breast haematoma

1. Introduction

A breast haematoma is a hematic collection within the breast tissue .

Often caused by trauma or surgery, or sometimes spontaneously in people on anticoagulant therapy. It may present as a palpable mass, with pain and sometimes a change in skin colour.

2. Etiology

Often caused by trauma or surgery, or sometimes spontaneously in people on anticoagulant therapy. It may present as a palpable mass, with pain and sometimes a change in skin colour.

3. Imaging

Breast haematoma imaging mainly ultrasound and sometimes mammography or MRI to assess the presence, size and nature of the haematoma.

On ultrasound, a haematoma may appear as a mass, circumscribed, anechoic or heterogeneous, depending on its stage development. Mammography and MRI can also help to assess the extent of the haematoma and distinguish this condition from other breast abnormalities.

Mammography can show a rounded mass with circumscribed contours, while MRI provides a detailed view of the characteristics of the haematoma, including its relationship with the surrounding breast structures.

4. References

1) Journo G, Bataillon G, Benchimol R, Bekhouche A, Dratwa C, Sebbag-Sfez D et al. Hyperechoic breast images: all that glitters is not gold! Insights Imaging 2018; 9: 199-209.

2) American College of Radiology. Illustrated breast imaging reporting and date system (BIRADS), 3rd edn. Reston: American College of Radiology, 2013.

3) Stavros AT, Thickman D, Rapp CI, Denis MA, Parker SH, Sisney GA. Solid breast nodules: use of sonography to distinguish between benign and malignant lesions. Radiology 1995; 196: 123-124.

4) Linda A, Zuiani C, Lorenzon M, Furlan A, Girometti R, Londero V et al. Hyperechoic lesions of the breast: not always benign. AJR 2011; 196: 1219-1224.

5) Linda A, Zuiani C, Lorenzon M, Furlan A, Londero V, Machin P et al. The wide spectrum of hyperechoic lesions of the breast. Clin Radiol 2011; 66: 559-565.

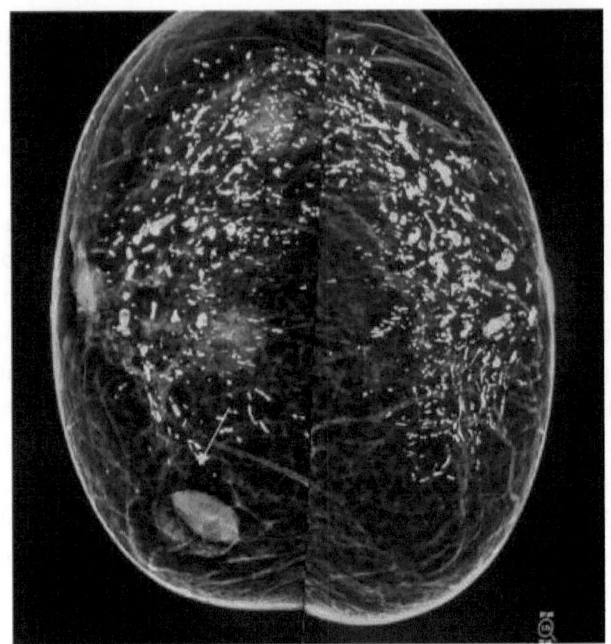

Figure 1: Bilateral mammogram. Oval breast mass on the right, with circumscribed contours, intermediate tone, gradations.

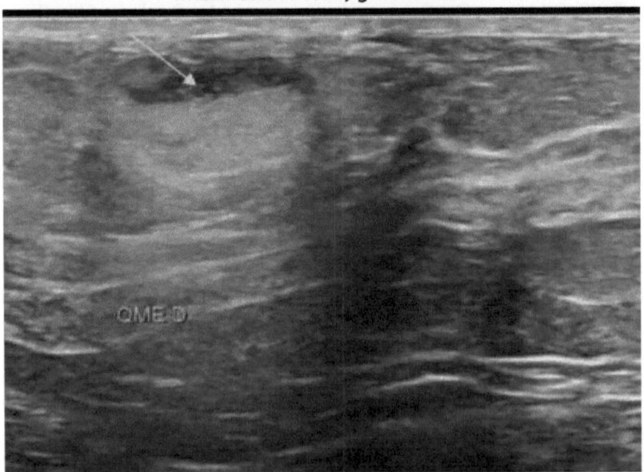

Figure 2. Breast ultrasound. Oval breast mass, with circumscribed contours, heterogeneous echogenic sarment of a liquid level

XVI. Intracanal papilloma

1. Introduction

Intraductal mammary papilloma is a benign tumour that develops within a milk duct, usually near the nipple. They may be solitary or multiple, particularly in young women (juvenile papillomatosis), asymptomatic or responsible for nipple discharge, sometimes bloody, which is the main clinical sign. The diagnosis of papilloma is based on histological study after biopsy or surgical removal. Breast imaging plays an important role in the detection, characterisation and follow-up of papillomas.

2. Imaging techniques

2.1. Mammography

> **Indications:** Initial detection, often following nipple discharge;

> **Technique:** Two standard views (cranio-caudal and medio-lateral oblique) are supplemented by additional views if necessary;

> **Results:** In the case of an intra-canal papilloma, mammography may show ductal dilatation, a mass or calcifications. However, papillomas are often too small to be detected by mammography alone.

2.2. Breast ultrasound

> **Indications:** Complementary evaluation, particularly useful for women under 40 or to evaluate the internal structures of masses detected on mammography;

> **Technique:** Use of high-resolution probes to examine areas of interest;

> **Results:** Can show ductal dilatation with or without an intraductal mass. The presence of vascularisation within the mass on the Doppler study is strongly suggestive of a papilloma.

2.3. Galactography

> A specific technique in which a contrast product is injected into the milk ducts. Papillomas are manifested by filling defects or irregularities in the ducts;

> **Indications:** Used symptoms such as suspicious nipple discharge are present.

2.4. Breast MRI

> **Indications**: Used for further evaluation when mammography and ultrasound results are inconclusive or to assess the extent of disease ;

> **Technique**: Acquisition of multiplanar sequences before and after gadolinium injection in T1 and T2 weighted sequences;

> **Results**: MRI can show a mass with contrast and associated ductal dilatation. It is particularly sensitive for detecting occult intraductal lesions.

3. Care and Support

> **Biopsy**: A needle biopsy under ultrasound or mammography guidance is crucial to confirm the diagnosis;

> **Surveillance**: Papillomas without atypia can be monitored, especially if they are asymptomatic;

> **Surgery**: Surgical excision is recommended for papillomas with atypia, symptoms, or to exclude an associated malignancy.

4. Conclusion

Intracanal papillomas represent a diagnostic challenge in breast imaging due to their variable presentation and potential association with more serious lesions. Careful evaluation using appropriate imaging techniques is essential for accurate diagnosis and appropriate management. Decisions regarding surveillance or surgical intervention should be made in consideration of the individual characteristics of the lesion and the patient's preferences.

5. References

1) Diana Hodorowicz-Zaniewska, Joanna Szpor and Pawel Basta, "Intraductal papilloma of the breast - management", Ginekologia Polska, vol. 90, no 2, 2019, pp. 100-103 (ISSN 2543-6767, PMID 30860277, DOI 10. 5603/GP. 2019. 0017, read online)

2) W. Al Sarakbi, D. Worku, PF Escobar and K. Mokbel, "Breast papillomas: current management with a focus on a new diagnostic and therapeutic modality", International Seminars in Surgical Oncology, vol. 3, no 1, 17 January 2006, p.1 (ISSN 1477-7800, PMID 16417642, Central
PMCID PMC1395317, DOI 10. 1186/1477-7800-3-1.

3) Tardivon A, Bazot M. Imagerie de la femme: coordination Marc Bazot et Anne Tardivon; Volume 1, Sénologie. Médecine Sciences Publications-Lavoisier; 2014.

4) Rosen PP, Hoda SA. Breast pathology: diagnosis by needle core biopsy. Lippincott Williams & Wilkins; 2010.

5) Lam WWM, Chu WCW, Tang APY, Tse G, Ma TKF. Role of Radiologic Features in the Management of Papillary Lesions of the Breast. Am J

Roentgenol. May 1, 2006;186(5): 1322-7.

6) Chung J, Lee WK, Cha E-S, Lee JE, Kim JH, Ryu YH. Shear-Wave Elastography for the Differential Diagnosis of Breast Papillary Lesions. PloS One. 2016;11(11): e0167118.

7) Sarica O, Uluc F, Tasmali D. Magnetic resonance imaging features of papillary breast lesions. Eur J Radiol. 1 March 2014;83(3): 524-30.

8) Daniel BL, Gardner RW, Birdwell RL, Nowels KW, Johnson D. Magnetic resonance imaging of intraductal papilloma of the breast. Magn Reson Imaging. 1 Oct 2003;21(8): 887-92.

9) Balu-Maestro C. Magnetic resonance imaging of the breast. J Radiol. 2001;82(1): 17- 26.

10) Park H-L, Kim LS. The Current Role of Vacuum Assisted Breast Biopsy System in Breast Disease. J Breast Cancer. March 2011;14(1): 1-7.

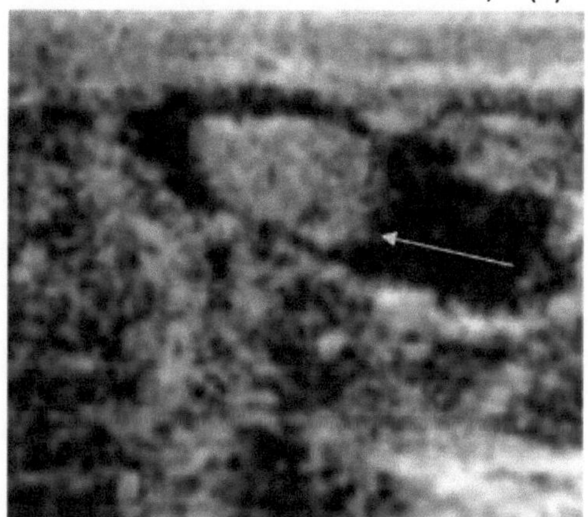

Figure 3: Mammary ultrasound: regular thin-walled retroareolar ductal ectasia with hypoechoic endo-canal content in relation to solitary papilloma.

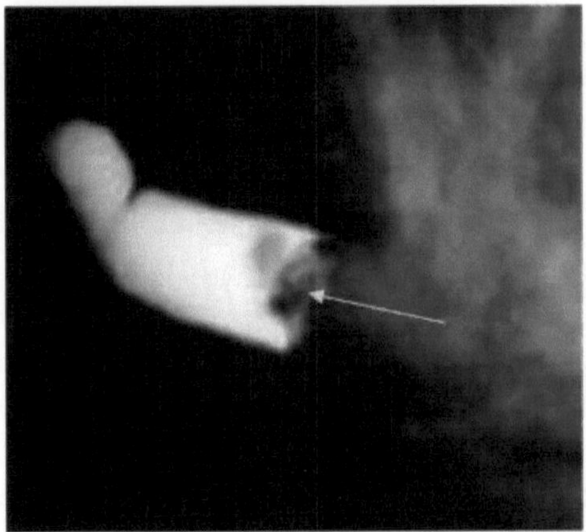

Figure 2: Galactography. Intraductal dilatation with a lacunar defect probably related to endo-canal displacement.

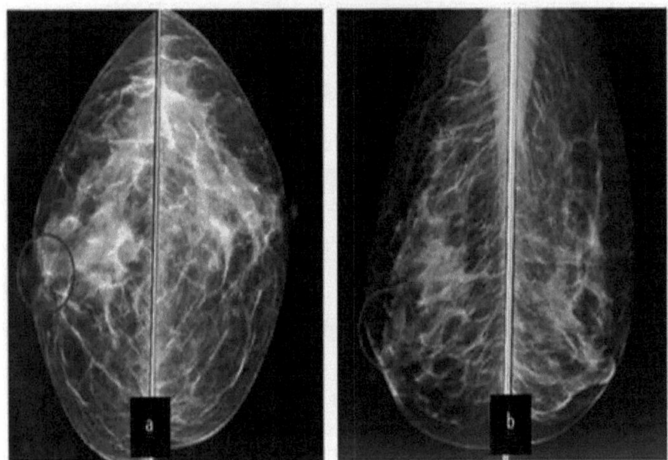

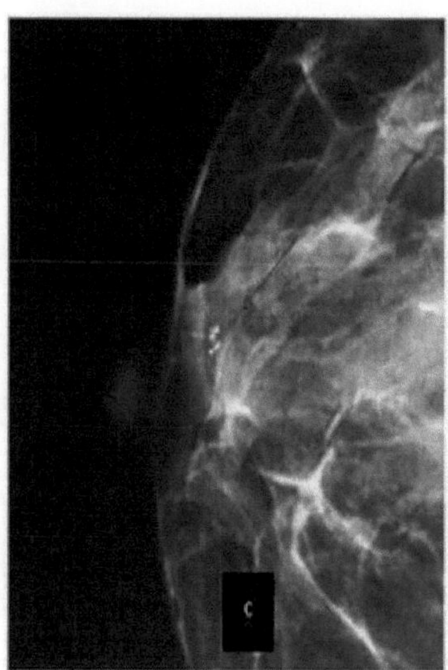

Figure 3. Bilateral mammogram, craniocaudal (a) and external oblique (b) views, magnification reveals a focus of coarse right retroareolar microcalcifications.

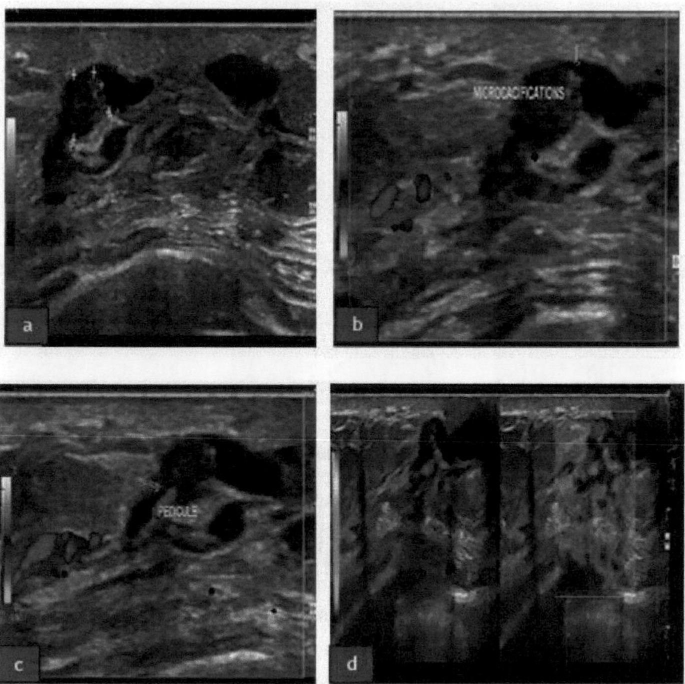

Figure 4. breast ultrasound (a) coupled with doppler (b, c) and elastography (d) Retroareolar ductal ectasia with a thin, regular wall and hypoechoic endo-canal content (a) containing microcalcifications (b), with a vascular pedicle (c), of intermediate consistency on elastography, associated with solitary papilloma.

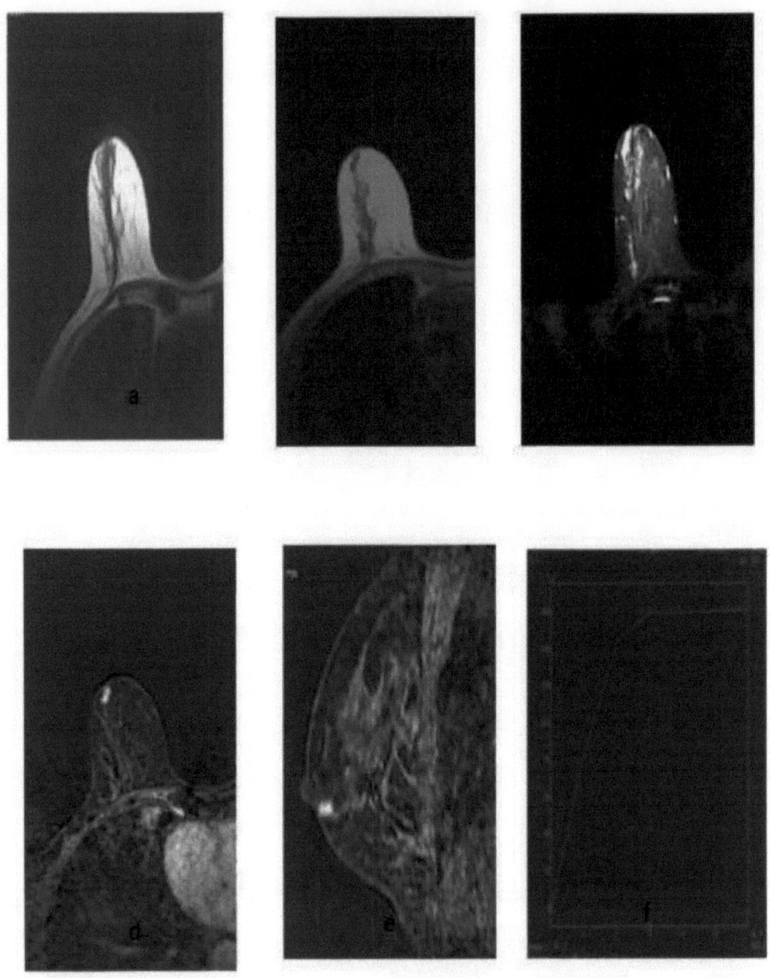

Figure 5. T1 (a), T2 (b), injected native (c) and subtracted (d) MRI of the breast. ductal ectasia, with thin, regular walls and nodular enhancement, homogeneous with a hemodynamic

homogeneous nodular enhancement with a type 2 haemodynamic curve

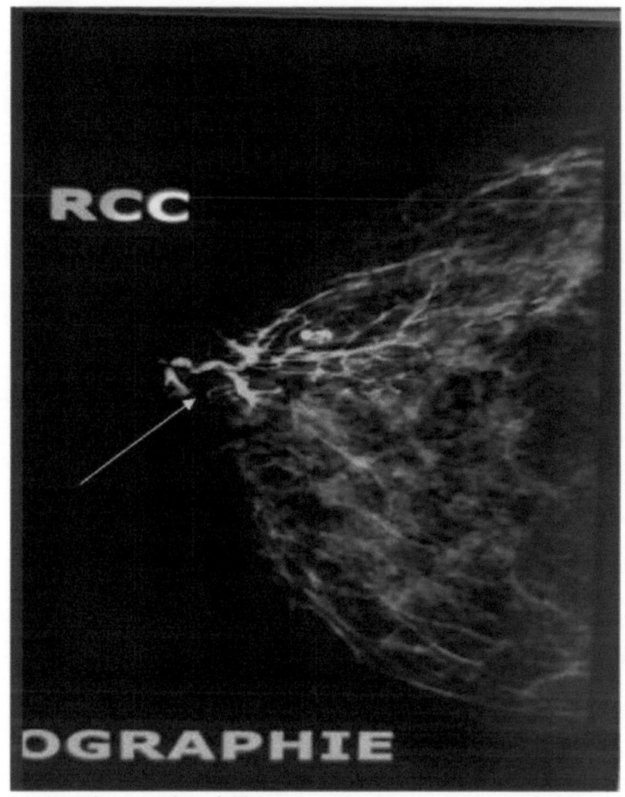

Figure 6: Galactography. Intraductal dilatation with a lacunar image probably related to endo-canal displacement.

XVII. Mammary cytosteatonecrosis

1. Introduction

Breast cytosteatonecrosis is a benign breast condition resulting from the necrosis of fatty tissue in the breast. It can occur after breast trauma, surgery or radiotherapy, leading to the formation of necrotic fat nodules. Over time, fibrous transformation may occur, calcifying in over 50% of cases. Fibrosis is mainly responsible for the distorted appearance. It can sometimes mimic malignant lesions on imaging, hence the importance a precise diagnostic approach.

2. Etiology

The main causes of cytosteonecrosis include physical trauma (shocks, injuries), breast surgery and radiotherapy. The condition can also occur spontaneously in women with large breasts or excessive breast fat.

3. Symptoms

> **Palpable mass:** firm nodule, often painful to the touch;

> **Changes to the skin surface:** The skin may become red, sometimes with a sensation of heat;

> **Discharge:** Rare, may occur if inflammation is severe.

4. Imaging techniques

4.1. Mammography

Radiological manifestations are varied, with radiolucent lesions surrounded by corona calcifications that change over time, characteristic of cytosteatonecrosis. Irregular masses, eggshell or coarse calcifications and areas of oily density are also found. It may resemble breast cancer.

4.2. Mammary ultrasound

> Hypoechoic masses with or without posterior acoustic shadowing, bordered by calcifications. The appearance may be complex, solid and cystic;

> Vascularity: Typically avascular on Doppler;

> It is usually located under the skin scar, which allows the diagnosis to be made.

4.3. Mammary MRI

> **Appearance:** Areas of variable signal in T1 and T2, with an absence of significant post-contrast enhancement in necrotic areas. Calcifications may not be well visualised;

> **Indications** : Used for difficult cases, where mammography and ultrasound do not allow adequate assessment.

5. Care and Support

> **Monitoring**: If cytosteatonecrosis is well characterised and asymptomatic, simple monitoring may suffice;

> **Biopsy**: A needle biopsy may be taken to confirm the diagnosis in cases of atypical features or suspected malignancy.

6. Conclusion

Breast cytosteatonecrosis can present a diagnostic challenge because of its radiological similarity to malignant lesions. Careful evaluation using multiple imaging modalities is often required to confirm the diagnosis and guide management. Understanding the specific imaging features and clinical context is essential to avoid unnecessary treatment and ensure optimal patient management.

7. Reference

1) Fouque O, Kind M, Boulet B, Brisse H, Kemel S, Genah I et al. Diagnostic strategy in the face of a fatty soft tissue tumour in adults. J Imag Diagn Interv 2018; 1: 265- 283.

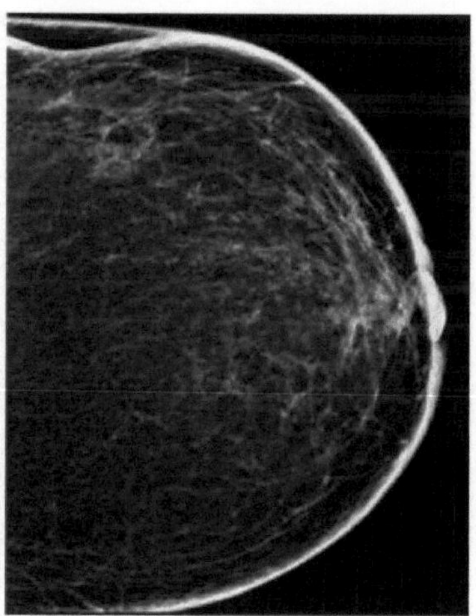
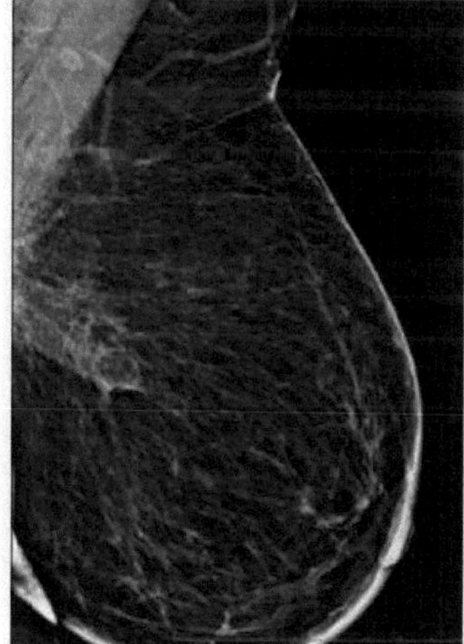

Figure 1: Front mammogram and left external oblique. Dense, heterogeneous, retractile area with sub-scarring clearness of the left QSE.

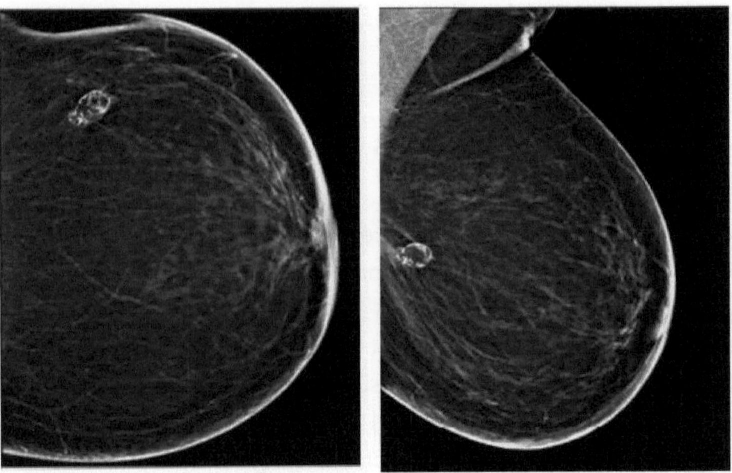

Figure 2 Mammogram, front and left external oblique. Progression over 2 years: Architectural distortion, retractile, dense, with calcified sub-scarring around the periphery, giving an eggshell appearance suggestive of a focus of cytosteato necrosis of the left breast fat.

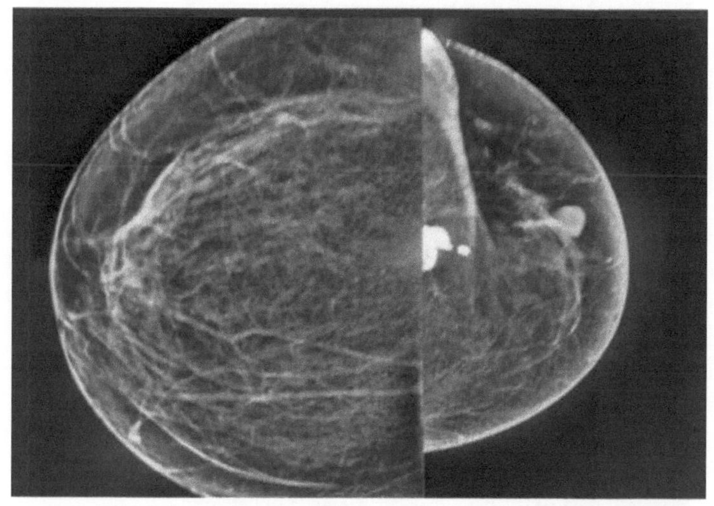

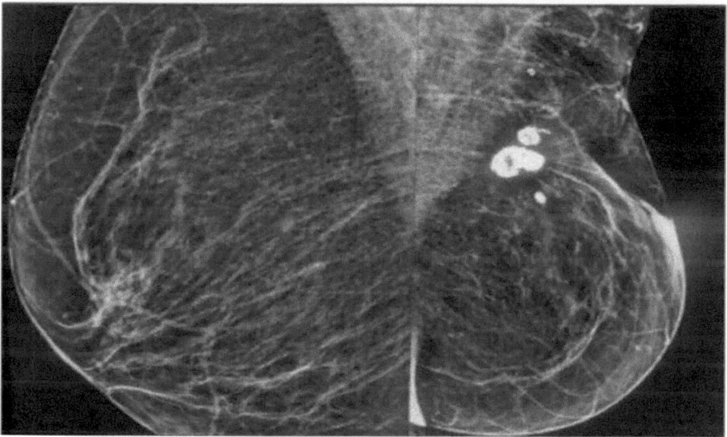

Figure 3: Bilateral frontal and external oblique mammograms. architectural distortion related to cicatricial retractile fibrosis deforming the contour of the dense, sub-scarred breast (lumpectomy), site of sub-scarred macro-calcifications, giving an appearance suggestive of a focus of cytosteato necrosis of the left breast fat.

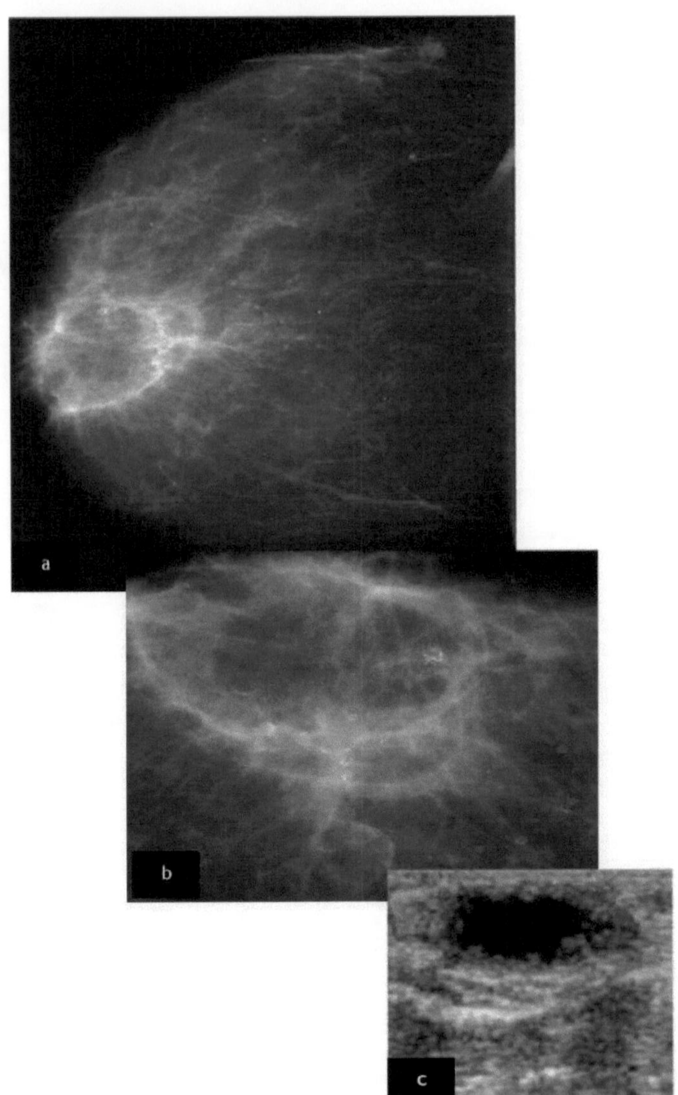

Figure 4: Front mammogram (a) and enlarged view (b): Peripheral calcified scarring, giving the appearance of an eggshell, a focus of cytosteato necrosis of right breast fat, (c) Breast ultrasound mimics a cyst with thick contents (echogenic +/- post enhancement.) non-attenuating (parietal calcifications).

XVIII. Pseudo angiomatous stromal hyperplasia

1. Introduction

Pseudoangiomatous hyperplasia (PAH) is a benign breast lesion characterised by a proliferation of blood ducts mimicking a vascular lesion, but consisting mainly of myofibroblastic tissue. Although it can occur at any age, it is more common in women of childbearing age and in menopausal women undergoing hormone replacement therapy, and can fluctuate in size with menstrual cycles.

2. Etiology

The exact cause of HPSA unclear, but it may be associated with trauma, surgery or inflammation of the breast. Hormonal changes also appear to play a role in its development. HPSA may be discovered incidentally during percutaneous sampling, when it is associated with other lesions (25% of percutaneous samples) or as an isolated tumour.

3. Imaging methods

3.1. Mammography

HPSA may not be visible on mammography or may appear as an asymmetric density with no specific features. Calcifications are rare. Limited characterisation of lesions, especially in dense breast tissue.

3.2. Mammary ultrasound

Several aspects have been described on ultrasound: hypoechoic mass with regular or blurred contours, more rarely hyperechoic. Generally, the most frequent appearance is that a hypoechoic mass, well limited, with or without apparent internal scarring. Central areas may appear more echogenic due to the presence of fibro glandular tissue.

Allows a detailed study of the internal structure of the lesion and guides biopsy if necessary.

3.3. Magnetic Resonance Imaging (MRI) of the breast

> MRI may show a lesion with intense, heterogeneous enhancement after injection of gadolinium, sometimes suggestive of a malignant lesion;

> Used in cases where the distinction between HSPA and a malignant lesion is not clear on other imaging modalities.

4. Differential diagnosis

> Breast carcinoma, particularly angiogenic forms;

> Hemangioma ;

> Fibroadenoma, in particular variants with myxoid changes ;

> Mondor disease (superficial thrombophlebitis of the breast).

5. Care and Support

> **Monitoring:** In most , HSPA can be monitored, particularly if the diagnosis is established with certainty and the lesion is asymptomatic;

> **Biopsy:** A biopsy may be necessary to exclude malignancy, particularly in the presence atypical features or rapid growth of the lesion;

> **Surgery:** Surgical excision is reserved for symptomatic cases, in cases of significant growth or if the diagnosis remains uncertain after biopsy.

6. Conclusion

Pseudoangiomatous stromal hyperplasia is a benign lesion of the breast that can present a diagnostic challenge due to its potential to mimic malignant lesions, particularly on MRI. A multimodal imaging approach is often required for accurate diagnosis. Knowledge of the distinctive radiological features of HSPA is essential to avoid unnecessary surgery and ensure appropriate patient management.

7. References

1) Brown AC, Audisio RA, Regitnig P. Granular cell tumour of thebreast. Surg Oncol 2011;20(2): 97-105.

2) Chen J, Wang L, Xu J, Pan T, Shen J, Hu W, et al. Malignantgranular cell tumor with breast metastasis: a case report andreview of the literature. Oncol Lett 2012;4(1): 63-6.

3) Yang WT, Edeiken-monroe B, Sneige N, Fornage BD. Appea-rances of granular cell tumors of the breast with pathologicalcorrelation. J Clin Ultrasound 2006;34(4): 153-60.

4) Scaranelo A, Bukhanov K. Granular cell tumour of the breast: MRI findings and review of the literature. Br J Radiol2007;80(960): 970-4.

5) Le BH, Boyer PJ, Lewis JE, Kapadia SB. Granular celltumor: immunohistochemical assessment of inhibin-alpha,protein gene product 9. 5, S100 protein, CD68, and Ki-67 proliferative index with clinical correlation. Arch Pathol LabMed 2004;128(7): 771-5.

6) Aoyama K, Kamio T, Hirano A, Seshimo A, Kameoka S. Gra-nular cell tumors: a report of six cases. World J Surg Oncol2012;10: 204.

7) Pergel A, Yucel AF, Karaca AS, Aydin I, Sahin DA, Demirbag N. A therapeutic and diagnostic dilemma: granular cell tumor ofthe breast. Case Rep Med 2011;2011: 972168.

8) Bowman E, Oprea G, Okoli J, Gundry K, Rizzo M, Gabram-Mendola S, et al. Pseudoangiomatous stromal hyperplasia(PASH) of the breast: a series of 24 patients. Breast J2012;18(3): 242-7.
9) Solomou E, Kraniotis P, Patriarcheas G. A case of a giant pseudoangiomatous stromal hyperplasia of the breast: magneticresonance imaging findings. Rare Tumors 2012;4(2): e23.
10) Virk RK, Khan A. Pseudoangiomatous stromal hyperplasia: anoverview. Arch Pathol Lab Med 2010;134(7): 1070-4.

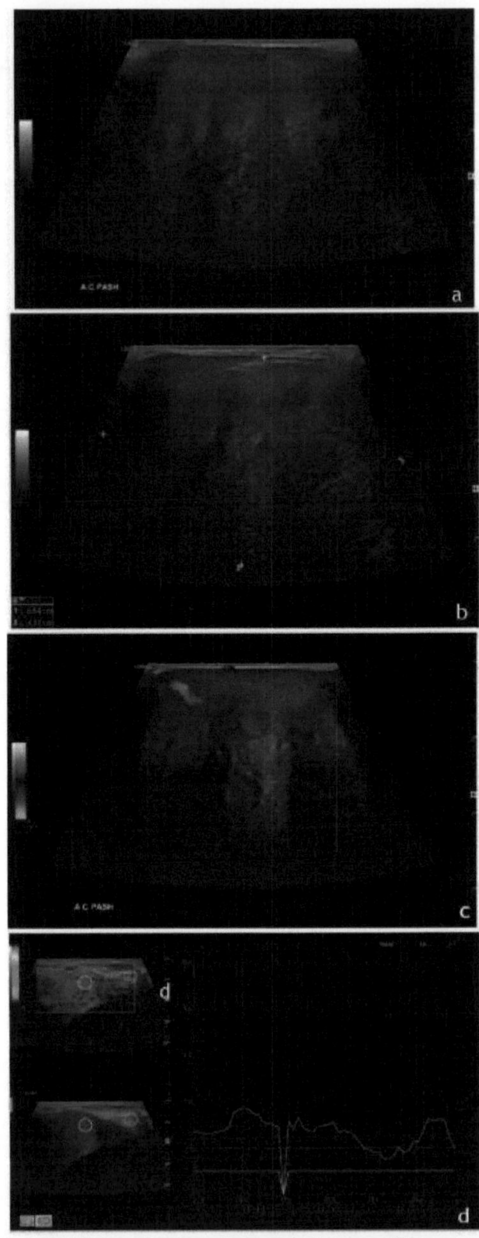

Figure 1: Breast ultrasound scan showing a hypoechoic mass with a roughly lobulated shape, circumscribed in places, indistinct in others, with fine echogenic spots, a long axis oblique to the cutaneous plane, measuring more than 7cm (Figure 2a, 2b), intermediate consistency on elastography (Figure 2c), and mixed vascularisation on colour Doppler (Figure 2d).

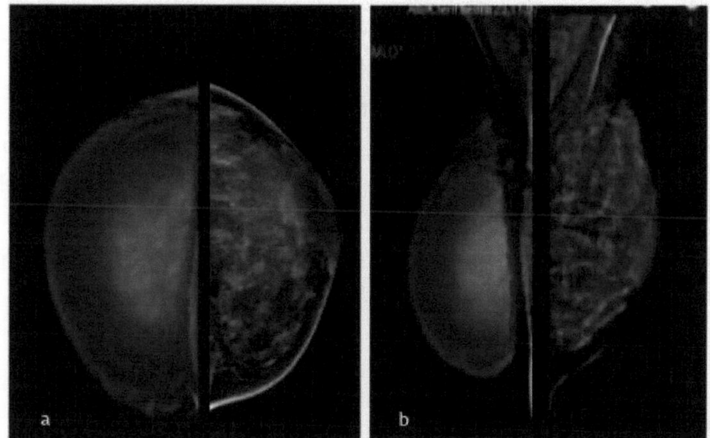

Figure 2: Bilateral mammogram *a. Craniocaudal view, b. External oblique view: Asymmetry of breast volume at the expense of the right breast with increased overall density without microcalcification.*

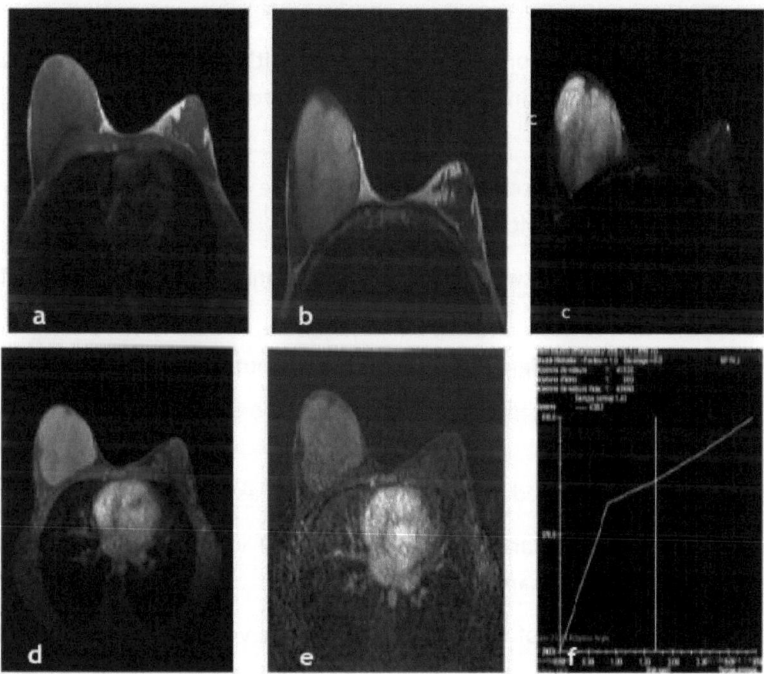

Figure 4: MRI of the breast, centred axial slices

a: T1 weighting; b: T2 weighting; c and d: T1 weighting with saturation of fat signal before and after gadolinium injection; e: subtraction sequence; f: type I enhancement curve. enhancement curve. Mass embedded in the gland in T2 hyposignal, T1 isosignal, with overall heterogeneous

heterogeneous enhancement.

XIX. Mondor disease

1. Introduction

Mondor disease is a superficial thrombophlebitis of the chest, usually of the thoracoepigastric vein. Although it can occur in both sexes, it is more common in women and may be associated with breast surgery, trauma or physical exertion.

Patients may experience pain, a hard palpable cord under the skin, and sometimes erythema along the affected vein pathway.

2. Medical Imaging

2.1. Ultrasound with colour Doppler

> **Indications :** Detection and assessment of thrombophlebitis ;

> **Technique:** Surface ultrasound with evaluation of blood flow in superficial veins;

> **Results:** May show a non-compressible vein with or without blood flow on Doppler evaluation, indicating the presence of a thrombus.

2.2. Mammography

> **Indications :** Rarely used for Mondor disease but can be performed to exclude other breast pathologies;

> **Technique:** Images in two standard views (craniocaudal and medio-lateral oblique);

> **Results:** No specific signs Mondor's disease, but useful for assessing the presence of breast masses or calcifications.

2.3. Breast MRI

> **Indications:** Can be used in complex cases or to assess complications;

> **Technique:** Multi-planar imaging in T1 and T2 weighted sequences, with contrast injection if necessary;

> **Results:** Visualisation of the superficial thoracic veins, enabling thrombosis to be identified.

3. Diagnosis

Is mainly clinical. Ultrasound is the technique of choice for confirming the diagnosis and ruling out other conditions.

4. Care and Support

Mondor disease is often self-limiting. Treatment may include anti-inflammatories, analgesics and hot compresses. In rare cases, anticoagulation may be necessary.

5. Conclusion

Mondor disease is a benign disorder with an excellent prognosis. Medical imaging plays a key role in diagnosis and helps to exclude other more serious conditions. A thorough understanding of the clinical presentation and imaging features is essential for accurate diagnosis and effective disease management.

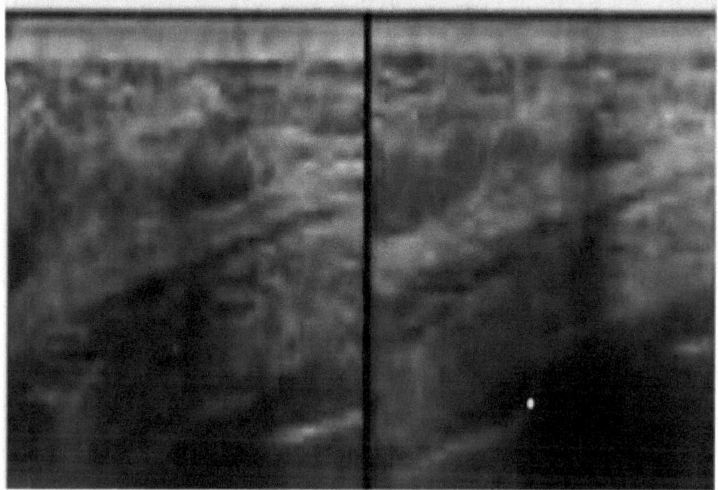

Figure. 1: Mammary ultrasound: anechoic elongated tubular structure with thin, regular walls finely echogenic, incompressible content, with no flow on the colour Doppler surrounded by a fine echogenic appearance of the surrounding fat suggestive of a superficial thrombosed vein.

superficial thrombosed vein.

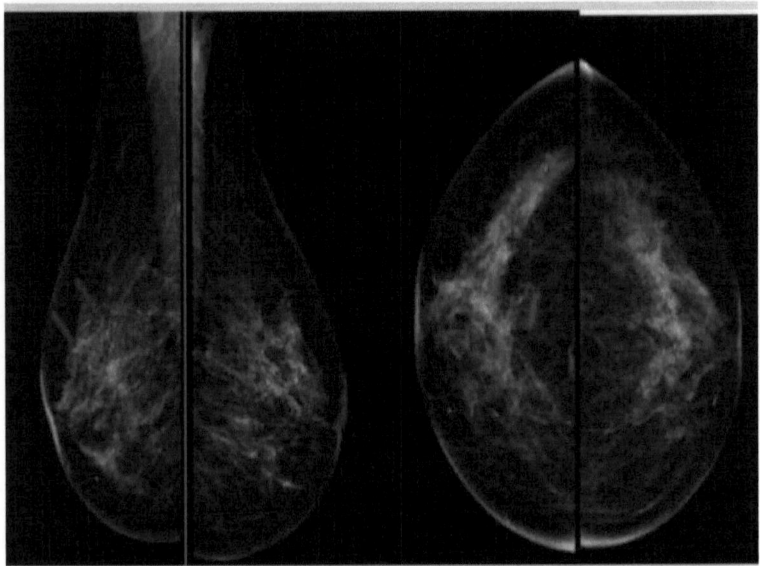

Figure 2. bilateral mammogram. Fine linear density along the path of the anomaly detected by ultrasound.

6. References

1) Fatnassi R, Kaabia O, Meski S, Ben Regaya L, Mkinini I, Briki R, Hidar S, Bibi M, Khairi H. Mondor disease of the breast. Imagerie de la Femme. 2009;19(4): 258-261.

2) Chiedozi LC, Aghahowa JA. Mondor's disease associated with breast cancer; surgery 1988;103: 438-9.

3) Quéhé P, Saliou AH, Guias B, Bressollette L. Mondor's disease: a case report. J Mal Vascul 2009;34: 54-60.

4) Kocaoglu M, Somuncu I, Ors F, Bulakbasi N, Tayfun C, Ucoz T. Imaging findings in breast involvement of Mondor's disease. European Journal of Radiology. 2004;52(3): 296-301.

5) Pugh CM, Dewitty RL. Mondor's disease. J Natl Med Assoc 1996;88: 359-63. [9] Hogan GF. Mondor's disease. Arch Intern Med 1964;113: 881-5.

6) Tournant B. Mondor's disease. In: Mastodynia. Le sein. Paris: Éditions ESKA; 2007 [p. 78-9]

7) Gokalp G, Mutlu H, Sonmez FC, Yildirim D, Kosar P, Kosar U. Mondor's disease of the breast: clinical, mammographic, and sonographic findings. European Journal of Radiology. 2008;66(3): 474-479.

8) Catania S, Zurrida S, Veronesi P, Galimberti V, Bono A, Pluchinotta A. Mondor's disease and breast cancer. Cancer 1992;69: 2267-70.

9) Hermann JB. Thrombophlebitis of breast and contiguous thoracoabdominal wall (Mondor's disease). NY State J Med 1966;15: 3146-52.

10) Gokalp G, Mutlu H, Sonmez FC, Yildirim D, Kosar P, Kosar U. Mondor's disease of the breast: clinical, mammographic, and sonographic findings. European Journal of Radiology. 2008;66(3): 474-479.

Conclusion

The discovery of benign lesions, even palpable ones, should no longer systematically refer patients to the surgeon. The radiologist is now the key player in the management of these lesions. there is a good clinical, radiological and histological match, there is little need for surgery.

Some indications for surgery are still unavoidable, given the risk of under-estimating pejorative lesions, which represent the limits of percutaneous techniques. In the future, improvements in these techniques and in histological diagnostics should further reduce these indications. The days of "remove first and think later" are definitely over!

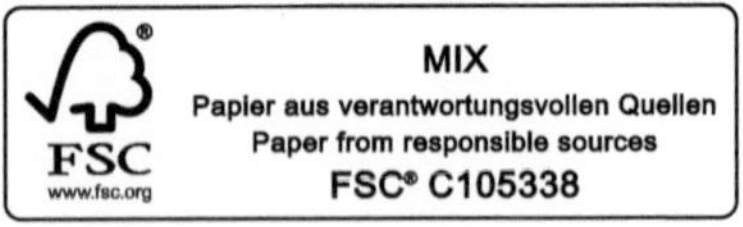

Printed by Books on Demand GmbH, Norderstedt / Germany